Caitlin Hildebrand, NP

Un-Less

Mindful Journaling for Body Positivity, Wellness & Unconditional Self-Love

Print ISBN: 978-1-09830-773-8

eBook ISBN: 978-1-09830-774-5

Acknowledgements

Thank you to my countless family, friends, colleagues and patients who have made this book possible. Your support, feedback, enthusiasm and love over a decade got me to this point of healing and sharing my story. You have helped me believe that we all deserve more, not less. Special thanks to my chiropractor, friend and photographer Dr Ed Camp, for your steadfast pursuit of creating the perfect images for the cover (and for healing my neck!). Endless love for my father, Derry Hildebrand, for being the best dad ever, and really listening and acknowledging how some family experiences fed into my eating disorder struggles. Lastly, to my husband and partner for almost sixteen years, John Turcik, thank you from the depths of my heart for your unwavering support of me, this book, and your consistent reinforcement of body positivity, wellness, and unconditional self love.

Table of Contents

PART I

Introduction

Do you struggle with how to nourish yourself? Do you over-eat or choose unhealthy processed foods, especially when stressed? Do you find yourself restricting or fearing what you eat, afraid of gaining weight? Do you have 30, 50, 100 extra pounds, or battle diabetes, heart disease, and other lifestyle related conditions? Do you obsess over what you eat and feel anxious or down if you miss a workout, or do you eat foods you consider taboo? These problems may seem in opposition to one another, but indeed they are just different manifestations of the same issue: a troubled relationship with food, body-image, and self-love.

This book is for all people, skinny and obese, normal weight and just plump, because almost all of us learned from an early age that food was love. We need to heal our relationships with food to really thrive, to have the healthy bodies, minds, and spirits we were born to have.

This book started as a blog I wrote because of my own fraught relationship with food, body-image, and weight. I was able to heal using what I know as a nurse practitioner (NP) and yoga and mindfulness teacher. Here, I will share with you my own journey, through Anorexia, Bulimia, and even obesity, and how I overcame my own unhealthy eating behaviors and became my most vibrant self through mindfulness journaling and unconditional self-care.

As an NP, I have the training, knowledge, and experience to help you understand the science and psychology behind poor self-care and nutrition. After many years of practice working with people who struggle with making change, I can how show you how to make modifications that really stick. Extensive research shows that journaling is one of the most successful interventions for people to sustain long-term behavior change, particularly regarding nutrition and activity.

Still, this is not a diet book. It is a book to guide you, using the proven tools of mindfulness, onto your own best path for wellness. It is a way to overhaul your relationship with yourself, so that when you eat and exercise, you do so to show yourself love. You will reach deep inside yourself to learn about your own triggers, needs, and joys, and only then will you begin to change how you eat and exercise. Through this rich process of exploration, you will create a new way of living that can bring you more longevity, wellness, and energy than you ever thought possible. Our bodies reflect our inner selves, and, as you heal within, you will begin to beam. Get ready for radiance in body, mind, and spirit.

Mindfulness and Behavior Change

Acclaimed mindfulness meditation researcher Jon Kabat-Zinn has defined mindfulness as "paying attention to the present moment, without judgment, and with loving kindness." In terms of meditation, this means tuning into the sensations in your own body, or, in the environment, to focus on the here and now, and to respond with tenderness and care. Can eating become meditation? Can we tune into our bodies to really listen to our own deep wisdom about how to best serve the body, mind, and spirit? How?

I believe that, in terms of changing eating behaviors and body-image to promote self-love, mindfulness means listening to your body, right now, regarding whether you are truly hungry and what nutrients, portions, and flavors would serve you best at this moment. That is mindful dining. But it is only part of it and, honestly, a small part of it. It is not the part that brings true wellness.

Many students of mindfulness have experienced the classic raisin experiment, where you very slowly eat a raisin, experiencing all the sensory components that we often ignore. Sometimes, meditation teachers also guide you to reflect on how the raisin was grown and made its way to you, as a method of honing awareness and gratitude about food production. These are valuable practices. Still, we cannot live our lives methodically eating raisins at a snail's pace. We need a way to eat in the real world and to do so with loving kindness not just in the moment, but in the long term. Only this can change our attitudes about food and body-image in a way that changes choices for the long haul.

Indeed, for eating, most people are already all about the now. We want what will taste best, right this minute; our brains and our cultural tendencies propel us to choose high sugar, high salt, and high fat foods. So, mindful dining is about more than focusing on the now. It is also about reflecting on the past and considering the future. It is about deep contemplation on how eating behaviors have affected us over time and are likely to impact our futures. This deep contemplation is not done easily from moment to moment, not in our fast-paced lives, which involve juggling work, family, and every other obligation and responsibility you can name. Mindful dining must hone a deep understanding to create habits that make the healthier choice the easy option that feels right. Every mouthful should not have to be a thoughtful choice. Through mindful self-reflection, you develop an awareness that is about more than the what, or the how, or the now. It is about the why.

One of my specialties is teaching quality improvement (QI), and all of my QI students will tell you that I always stress that to create buy-in, you have to lead with the Who and the Why. I did not develop this: I instead learned it from Simon Sinek's "Golden Circle"

TedTalk.[1] He emphasizes that to create change, you have to lead with the why. The same goes with creating your own change toward better health. Why do you want to run a 5K? Why do you want to lose 20 pounds? If the answer is to look better on Friday night, you will probably very quickly find another thing more important to focus on—because pretty much everything thoughtful people care about is more important than how you look on a Friday night. Instead, if your reason is to lose weight to promote your fertility so you can have a family, or to eat better to reduce your risk of cancer that runs in your family, then, and really only then, will you sustain focus and make the choices that predict change for the long term.

Start with your why. Why are you reading this book? Pause. Really answer it. Why, of all the zillion books out there, did you decide to read this book on using mindful self-reflection to heal your relationship with food and your body-image? Was it to fit into a bridesmaid's dress you ordered too tight? That's doubtful. It is probably about something much deeper than what the scale can tell you (which is minimal). It is probably because you have spent many hours beating yourself up, either by bingeing, purging, restricting, or simply admonishing yourself for what seemed like a good decision at the time, for failed "solutions" you have tried, for problems you thought you had.

When I struggled with bulimia, making myself vomit felt like a solution. It made me feel like I was in control. I felt bloated and panicked after overeating, and, although I knew it was unhealthy, I could justify it because I did not do it all the time. We humans are expert at justification.

---

1   Simon Sinek, "How Great Leaders Inspire Action," September 2009, Newcastle, Wyoming. TED video, 17:50, https://www.ted.com/talks/simon_sinek_how_great_leaders_inspire_action?language=en

When I struggled with anorexia, restricting calories in an attempt to lose weight felt like a solution. It made me feel like I was in control. I felt chubby, and cutting calories seemed like the way to look in the mirror and be able to love myself and to be loved as a ballerina and as a young woman. I knew it was not healthy to obsess over my weight. Still, I could justify it because I was still able to dance and get good grades, which I thought showed I must be well-nourished enough. It was not until I was so dizzy that I had to lie down during dance class and constantly left class to urinate (from bingeing on water to inhibit hunger), that I acknowledged that my obsessions were actually controlling me.

Many years later, when I struggled with obesity, eating whatever sounded delicious, at whatever portion I desired, also felt like a solution. It made me feel like I was in control. It felt like a way to break free from the social and cultural norms that told me a woman is only valuable if she looks and acts a certain way. It made me feel carefree and relaxed. Until I looked at pictures and hardly recognized myself. Until I tried to hike Yosemite, and my knees ached, and I could not keep up with my friends.

In other words, when you are trying to solve the wrong problem, you will come up with all kinds of wrong solutions. Through all these unhealthy patterns, I was trying to solve the problem of feeling worthy. Deep down, I have always feared that I am not worthy of self-love just as I am. Not worthy of love, unless, unless, unless. There was always a condition.

Thankfully, I grew up in a home full of love. My family never made me suffer. Although food and weight were constantly discussed, which was not a healthy obsession, my family never made me feel as though my real worth depended on the number on the scale. As imperfect as my family's focus on dieting was, unfortunately most people grow up in far worse environments. The Adverse Childhood Experiences study of over 15,000 people done by Kaiser Permanente Healthcare and the Centers for Disease Control (CDC) showed us that early childhood traumas are extremely common, and these set people up for dramatically higher risks of health problems, from cancer and obesity to lung disease and suicide.[2] It is not surprising that the more exposure to abuse, neglect, substance abuse, and mental illness people have, the more likely they are to make poor health choices. They develop a hair-trigger stress response in their sympathetic nervous system that hardwires them to over-produce stress hormones to normal life stressors. Their bodies go into fight or flight with a simple disagreement, and they either lash out or crash inwards. Many times, especially in women, this manifests as self-harm that is hard to see and which may be small and cumulative. Snorting coke is easy to identify as self-abuse, but drinking a liter of Coke every day to stay energetic when you're chronically run-down is not. Neither is beating yourself up emotionally when you drink a single Coke and obsessing over how to burn off the calories.

This is why it is critical to know your why. Most people aren't harming themselves when they drink a Coke once in a while. And no one intends to. However, if you already have diabetes or heart disease, over time you will. Of course, no single behavior is particularly harmful, or even healthy. Truly, only patterns are. Exercising is only healthy when done in moderation. So is kale. We can abuse ourselves with too much or too little. Too often or too rarely. That is why the *why* is so crucial. Knowing your why is what teaches you what you need.

---

2   Felitti et al., "Relationship of childhood abuse and household dysfunction to many of the leading causes of death in adults," *American Journal of Preventive Medicine* 14, no. 4 (May 1998): 245-258.

Even with my many years' experience as a nurse practitioner and yoga and mindfulness teacher, I cannot diagnose your true problem, and I cannot prescribe your true why. I cannot tell you how to define what true wellness is for you: how much to eat, what to eat, how to move, or when. Only you can learn that from your own mindful reflection. It is totally individual. That is why self-reflection is the key to wellness. Mindfulness is a key component in building that self-awareness. Thankfully, how to ask yourself what you need can indeed be taught; I believe mindful journaling for wellness is the best way to do that.

So, what is mindful journaling for wellness? First, let's talk about what it's not. It's not writing a rant about why you hate your belly. It's not about methodically tracking your activity or your calories. It is not about labeling foods good or bad or labeling body parts as good or bad. Unconditional wellness involves letting go of good and bad altogether. Mindfulness derives from Buddhism, and a key principle of Buddhism is non-attachment. Non-attachment is not about not caring. It is about letting go of the struggle: the struggle for more, the struggle for less, and the attachment to the outcome. If you are reading this book because you believe you will happier 30 pounds less, I hate to break it to you, but you won't be. You might look slimmer and be able to fit into clothes you like more, but if you don't do the work to let go of defining happiness based on how you look, you will never be satisfied.

I, like most everyone on earth, don't love my belly hanging over my jeans. Still, my journey through anorexia, bulimia and obesity have taught me one very crucial lesson. You will not be happier skinnier. I will say it again. You will not be happier skinnier. What makes people feel happier is feeling inspired, appreciated, creative, and feeling like they matter. The only way to do that is to invest yourself deeply in your why. Sure, healthy eating and being active are crucial for optimal physiological health, but they will not bring happiness if they are conditional: that is, if you only tell yourself that you are good enough *when*... beautiful when. Real wellness is unconditional.

So, how do you develop a self-love that is unconditional, and how do you tie this to making choices that enhance wellness? Well, first we must define wellness. Wellness is not a size. Wellness is not fitness. Wellness is holistic mind, body, and spirit radiance. It is about feeling at peace with yourself and your life, even when things around you may be chaotic, when your past may be full of suffering, and when your future may be uncertain. That is where mindfulness comes in. Mindfulness helps you to focus on the here and now, to let go of 15 minutes ago or 15 years ago, when your co-worker made you feel stupid, your mother made you feel unwanted, or your daughter made you feel unappreciated. It brings you into this moment—and to the possibility of a better future—through simply being in the now. It respects that whatever you do right now will impact the future. Being mindful helps you avoid acting on subconscious impulses that lead you away from your goals.

Similarly, motivational interviewing is a model of coaching in which a guide helps you clarify your goals and design self-directed plans to achieve them. Central to motivational interviewing is the principle that people believe what they themselves say. So, through guided journaling, this book prompts motivational self-interviewing. You will literally write your own book for wellness.

When you eat with mindfulness, you ask yourself the real questions that help you solve the real problems. The real question is not whether that Snickers bar has "too many" calories. (It doesn't. No one candy bar will have any impact whatsoever.) The real question is more likely this: will eating it make you feel better physically, mentally, or emotionally? Only you will know. Sometimes it may, sometimes it may not. I cannot tell you. I can only teach you how to ask yourself. And when you learn to ask yourself, you learn to solve the real problems and get to the real solutions that will free you from conditional self-love. You will learn that wellness is about letting go of the belief that you are less, that you are not beautiful already, perfect already. Real wellness is about creating unconditional self-love that drives self-care. Wellness is not about less of anything, at least not all of the time. It is *un-less*. It is only about more. More acceptance, more compassion, more space, more clarity, more love. Wellness is about caring for yourself because you are sacred and deserve more, not less.

My Story

When I was young, I watched all the adults in my life struggle with their weight. They tried practically every diet: Jenny Craig, Weight Watchers, McDougall, Medi-Fast, you name it. They all "worked"—they all helped my family members lose weight if they could stick to them. But none of them delivered what they promised: well-being. Why? Because none of them even touched on the underlying problem. My family used food to soothe, and diets are about the least soothing thing possible. My family knew all about good nutrition. A lack of knowledge was not the issue. They had demanding careers and a big family to support, so stress was never-ending. When tired, irritated, or dealing with any other unpleasant feeling, they ignored their nutritional knowledge and made unhealthy choices. Usually for them, this was in terms of portion size. As we all know, you can have too much of a good thing. In addition, they used food to celebrate, and, thankfully, we had a lot to celebrate. Eating was about far more than hunger. In sum, my family was obsessed with health, and yet they were unhealthy. Their work and obligations trumped everything else. Wellness and being active was always the lowest priority.

As a result, I watched my parents yo-yo diet throughout my childhood and adolescence, losing and gaining weight, gaining and losing self-esteem. Therefore, when I started puberty and gained some weight (a normal healthy amount for my development), I thought I needed to diet too. Also, I was a dancer, and I spent hours each day looking in the mirror, scantily clad, comparing myself to the very thin older ballerinas I idolized.

When I was about ten, my father started following the McDougall diet, a very low fat, high carb, vegetarian diet. I began to follow it too, and, as an animal lover, it was easy to get behind the cruelty-free philosophy. However, it also became a way for me to eliminate entire food groups and not have people question me. Many people who make major food changes in the name of health or other principals can be subconsciously doing the same thing: finding a way to control intake while flying under the radar.

When I was just beginning junior high, we moved from a small town in Northern California to a major city in Southern California. There, I entered a much more competitive ballet school, and I was surrounded by a culture obsessed with youth and looking good. Even more importantly, my mother and the nanny who had raised me had a major falling out. I was not allowed to see or speak to my nanny. I was struggling with my own development as a woman, adjusting to a new place, and wanting to please everyone around me. As a bright student in a very driven family, I had always been a perfectionist, but it took on a new level of obsession. I was, in all, the perfect candidate for an eating disorder.

I knew I was not overweight, but I wanted to be slimmer. I made a food and exercise journal, often threw away food, and drank copious amounts of water. I lost weight, about 25 pounds, at exactly the time I should have been growing. I was totally obsessed, reading every diet book and article I could get my hands on. I remember calculating that out of every hour, I spent 20 minutes thinking about "health," though this was probably a gross underestimate. I was far from healthy, though: I was usually dizzy, my bones hurt when I lay down, and I developed the excess body hair called *lanugo* associated with anorexia. Unfortunately, my parents seemed to think I was just acting like any other serious dancer. The closest my mother got to recognizing the problem was taking me to the doctor because I was urinating so much. He just told me I was drowning myself from the inside out and missed the entire pattern of eating disorder symptoms.

On some level, though, I myself recognized there was a problem. A fellow dancer and I made a pact not to let ourselves go below 90 pounds. I still remember this conversation vividly because it showed just how troubled I was. I became focused on eating disorders, accusing friends of having them and creating a science project about social pressures and eating disorders in dancers that went all the way to state science fair. Still, I did not recognize that I needed help. However, when I see pictures of myself then, all bones and sunken cheeks, I shudder. Moving back to my small town at the beginning of high school helped, but I continued to struggle.

When I was about 16, I quit ballet after recognizing that my body image and mental health were really fraught. Although I loved dancing, I knew I could not be healthy surrounded by a culture that celebrates such a gaunt aesthetic. One lauded choreographer, Balanchine, is famous for saying he wanted to see every bone in a dancer's body! I loved to dance, but I was suffering deeply and knew

I could not sustain myself when obsessed with weight and constantly anxious.

I went back to gymnastics, which I had done as a young child. I was drawn to rhythmic gymnastics, a graceful form in which you dance and tumble while using ribbons, hoops, clubs, etc. My coach stressed fun and never mentioned weight. She herself ate a balanced diet and encouraged us to do the same. She wanted us to look strong, not thin. I began to relax about what I ate. She was realistic about our goals, knowing it was just a hobby. I started having a normal social life, including a boyfriend who made me feel beautiful.

Eventually, on my seventeenth birthday, I even gave up being a vegetarian. Though I absolutely still think vegetarianism is the kindest way to treat animals, this change was a healthy sign for me. It indicated that I was no longer so rigid about food. I was no longer living by rules. I was starting to eat for joy.

Still, in college, like many others, I gained some weight. I was no longer in a consistent sport, and I drank alcohol frequently, causing me to fill out. For me, this was mostly in my chest, and people even asked me if I had gotten a breast enlargement when I came home for winter break. Indeed, in some ways, I was really just finishing the puberty my body had been starved from accomplishing.

Over the years, I continued to gain weight very slowly. I would occasionally make myself vomit, and I intermittently tried diet pills. Overall, however, I did not exhibit any debilitating patterns. From the outside, I looked like a totally normal young woman, but, on the inside, I felt quite anxious about my new-found curves. I tried to eat healthily and worked out mostly for fitness, but, by the time I finished college, I was a bit overweight. I moved in with my boyfriend, whom I then married soon after. He was a wonderful host, who loves to celebrate and embraces eating for pleasure. Unfortunately, this led me to eat and drink as he did, with plenty of wings, pizza, and alcohol. Indeed, I was also actually afraid to try to lose the weight, because I feared I could trigger my eating disorder again. I felt trapped. I then developed some severe digestive problems, which lead me to lose some weight rapidly. It was almost a high for me to lose weight, which shows how fraught I still was. But after I healed, I gained all the weight back and more.

I decided to speak to a therapist about my occasional purging, and she led me to a breakthrough. She pointed out that when I made myself throw up because I felt guilty and bloated from overeating, all it did was make me feel guiltier. It compounded how awful I felt. Recognizing that the purging made me feel worse, not better, helped me let it go. I haven't thrown up since.

Still, in 2008, my body mass index went into the obese category, and I started to worry. (Body mass index, or BMI, is a tool for measuring height-to-weight ratio. Although it is imperfect, especially for those with significant muscle mass, and waist-to-hip ratio is better, it is a commonly used barometer for healthy weight.) As a new registered nurse, I wanted to project a healthy example for my patients. Even more importantly, I was determined to avoid all the chronic diseases associated with obesity, like diabetes, cardiovascular disease, and many cancers. How could I get to a healthy size without risking my mental health?

One marker of eating disorders is secrecy, so I knew that if I wanted to slim down in a healthy way, I would have to be honest about what I was doing. I would need friends and family to monitor my actions and give me feedback. I decided to blog. At the time, my goal was just to get down to a normal-weight BMI, which for my height is 143 pounds. When I was a teenager, "143" was pager code for "I love you," so from a chance coincidence came the central concept of my plan: self-love.

The blog was a terrific success. It was far more than a food journal, which typically includes simply what you eat and weigh. I also reflected upon my triggers, as well as my observations about body image, health, and wellness. Many friends, family members, and even co-workers read it and gave me support. When I started to get a little obsessive, one friend, a nurse on the eating disorders unit at the psychiatric hospital where we worked, would remind me to be more flexible and kinder to myself. It was a healing practice, to publicly examine my own relationship with food and exercise. I learned to eat well and be active, not within a framework of deprivation, but of self-care. I centered my eating on natural whole foods, with abundant fruits and vegetables and protein, and I limited sugar and alcohol. I loved the process of blogging, and my readers encouraged me to start writing this book.

Over about six months, I lost over thirty pounds, and I was vibrant and happy. Eventually, though, I was at a healthy weight, but I found myself making choices, such as limiting my portions, not because it was appropriate, but because I knew others would be reading the blog. It had become something with the potential to cause harm—to lead me to not listen to my own hunger or intuition. So, I stopped writing. It was the right choice at the time. Using the general principles of the plan, I then maintained my size for about five years.

This started to change after I began eating dairy products. I had avoided them since 2008, when eliminating them had fixed my digestive issues. However, in 2013, I tested my sensitivity and found I had healed. I then went back to being mostly vegetarian, and I was soon eating a diet centered on cheese and processed carbs: pasta, pizza, etc. I was never obese again, but the weight crept up. I was what we shall call "pleasantly plump": overweight but not technically at risk for disease. Indeed, that is the medical definition for the difference between being overweight and being obese. Being overweight means you have some excess body fat, but being obese means the fat has reached a level of danger, mainly because of the way adipose (fat) cells create inflammation in the body, which is a central feature of most disease.

I have bachelor's and master's degrees from the University of Pennsylvania, as well as national certification and licensure as an Adult and Geriatric Nurse Practitioner since 2011. This allows me to diagnose disease and prescribe treatment. I have extensive experience treating severe chronic illness, most of which is associated with poor nutrition and inactivity. As a primary care provider for primarily low-income, frail elders, I have focused my career on serving people struggling with the end results of many years of poor self-care, such as blindness and amputations due to end stage diabetes, kidney failure, advanced lung disease, and recurrent strokes and heart attacks. I have also cared for numerous people contending with substance abuse and mental health issues, many of whom battle obesity as a result of using food and alcohol as a way to self-soothe.

My own minor excess weight was, quite appropriately, not notable in the face of the severe chronic disease I saw every day. Still, as time went on and the responsibility and stress piled up, I was neglecting my own needs. I ate whatever seemed okay and exercised inconsistently. Then, in 2014, my mother was diagnosed with terminal pancreatic cancer. It took all my energy to care for her, my family, and my patients. Surprisingly, doing a second master's in Health Administration helped me focus on a positive thing I could succeed in. Still, I was giving far more than I could to stay balanced.

Feeling overwhelmed, I started using an antidepressant, bupropion, which helped enormously with the apathy and irritability that came with caregiving and worry. Thankfully, this medication, unlike many other anti-depressants, is not associated with weight gain. This, as well as therapy, helped me get through a critical time without using food as a coping mechanism—in other words, I did not overeat, nor did I restrict. Indeed, in the hardest time of my life, I managed not to use food to manage my stress. For someone with a history of eating disorders, this healthy result during a period of severe suffering is really rather rare. I credit self-love principles for giving me the perspective that allowed me to cope constructively.

About a year after my mother died, I felt determined not to ever have to tell my own family I had a disease related to poor self-care. (Being obese was my mother's only risk factor for this extremely lethal form of cancer). I finished my second master's degree with top grades and was chosen as graduation speaker by my classmates. I took a job leading a home health and hospice company, and I improved the quality of care and loved my staff. I was very stressed, but I took fairly good care of myself, exercising regularly at the gym across the street from my office. Convenience is a key factor in making healthy choices! However, I realized after about six months that I was not ready for that level of stress and needed more mentorship. I boldly listened to my heart, quit, and took a new job with the Veterans Health Administration. This offered less direct power but more opportunity for growth and the chance to help vulnerable people who really needed me. Thankfully, I was able to spend a few months reflecting and really letting myself relax after a few years of intense stress. It was the best gift I could ever have given myself. I travelled a lot and ate and drank many fabulous local specialties. I was happy and enjoying all the world had to offer. I was able to taper down and then stop my antidepressant without any of the blues I feared.

After a couple months of travelling, though, I felt bloated and lackluster. I realized I wanted to start a new phase of life more centered and healthy. I had already started doing yoga almost every day since being in India, but I recognized I could really use an overall re-set of my wellness plan before beginning my new job. I decided to formally restart the eating approach I had developed with the blog, and I began writing a post every day focusing on wellness.

After visiting some family members who are great mentors for longevity and wellness, I concluded it was time to share my approach with the world. I gave myself the lofty goal of writing a book and finishing a draft before I began yoga teacher training a month later. Once I sat down to write, it quickly poured out of me. It is my way of life; I just needed to verbalize it. I shared drafts right away with beloved friends, especially those who work in healthcare and who have struggled with eating disorders and self-care. I wanted to see how the plan resonated with them. I got immense positive and constructive feedback. I credit their support to my faith that this approach is not just mine, but belongs to all of us.

Becoming a yoga teacher was a dream I had been delaying for years. Yoga allowed me to reconnect in a new way with choreography and movement, without significant focus on weight. I also completed training with the Center for Mind-Body Medicine and began leading mindfulness groups to help people manage stress and pain and improve their own self-care. Over time, I became even more invested in holistic wellness and combining evidence-based complementary and alternative modalities with conventional medicine. I am now a Fellow in Integrative Medicine with the University of Arizona and a Nurse Practitioner and Nurse Manager in our Integrative Health

Service at the VA. (Of note, the content of this book is my personal and professional opinion, and I am required to specify that the VA does not officially endorse it).

Now, as an NP and a yoga and mindfulness teacher, both for VA staff and in the community, I have even more reason to be a role model, physically and spiritually. I take it as a sign that everyone who has seen my evolution tells me how natural a fit it is. I am vibrant, strong, and energetic, and I feel comfortable in my own skin. I nourish myself holistically. I let go of the seduction of the diet mentality, setting myself free to follow my natural instincts and my intuition, key to the heart of yoga. I have revised the book to focus on what has helped me the most—mindfulness—which empowers us to really listen in to our internal wisdom, to give ourselves loving-kindness and unconditional love.

In all, I have poured out all I have lived, loved, and learned in this book. I have taken the risk of sharing my own story to show you the value of self-knowledge. I want you to know that I struggle just as you are struggling, but that the pain of getting to know your own darkness can bring light in the end. I am here to be your guide, to make suggestions, and to be a beacon of safety and encouragement and honesty. This book will teach you my story, as a person and as a healer, but you will write your own story and make your own plan. You will develop your own philosophy of wellness that is not limited, that is Un-Less.

Beginning Your Journey, Your Journal

Chances are, you might be tempted at this point to flip straight to the principles of Un-Less and start to try to change your behaviors. Please don't. Indeed, that is exactly what you should not do, unless you want to end up exactly where you started. You cannot learn which behaviors you could benefit from changing until you get to know yourself in a new way. Un-Less is not a quick fix, and that is not where the magic lies. The beauty is instead within the beholder: inside of you. You are the magic you need to learn to conjure.

The backbone of Un-Less is journal writing, so don't wait: go get a journal, or use the space on these pages. Start by using the reflection cues at the end of each section to inspire your digestion of the concepts. Jot down passages you find especially inspiring or even those that strike a nerve. Whatever these are, they are important for you to reflect on. Also, write down facts that you didn't know. If you like, draw, doodle, or make flow charts. I recommend hand-writing because it tends to promote retention, open-mindedness, and is less likely to feel like work. However, you can certainly type or even text parts of your journal, too. For the longer reflections, be sure to use the mode that will allow you to write most quickly and with the least interference, which will add to your depth. Don't worry about grammar. No one will read this except you, and it is not meant to be a finished product, just a way to shine light into darkness. Just let it flow. Start with the first word that comes to mind, and go from there.

Anytime you find yourself thinking about your body, eating, food, fitness, anything related to body-image, write in your journal. Before you begin, spend a minute or so focusing on your breath. This will help center you; breathwork, called *pranayama* in yoga, is a valuable tool because it is always available to you, it is free, and it can be done without anyone else knowing.

Before journaling, begin with slow, deep diaphragmatic breathing. This form of "soft belly" breathing, allows the abdominal muscles to relax and release. It stimulates the tenth cranial nerve, the vagus nerve, which connects the diaphragm to the brain, heart, lungs, and other main organs. The vagus nerve activates the parasympathetic nervous system, which creates the relaxation response. This is the rest and digest, tend and befriend mode, the antidote to the fight, flight, or freeze mechanism that is the stress response. The relaxation response boosts your calming neurotransmitters and, when used consistently, can even decrease stress hormones and, therefore, inflammation. Let your exhale be longer than your inhale; ideally, it should be twice as long, such as four counts in and eight counts out. Focus on the sensations of the breath: where you notice it, where it feels smooth and full. Really feel the feeling of it. Taking time to deep breathe before you journal cultivates psychological and physiologic calm within yourself. This will allow you to be more creative and less reactive—more mindful.

Once you have centered on the sensations of your breath, then envision yourself in the future, unconditionally well—vibrant, strong, joyful. Visualizing yourself in this way will help you come to regard your wellness in terms of power and energy. Just as elite Olympians use imagery to envision themselves clearing the high jump, you too can use imagery to envision yourself in your most vibrant state. Try to let go of any default expectations you might be carrying about what "health" looks like, the aesthetics of it. Health is a loaded word that for many people is associated with weight. Instead, focus on wellness, as defined not by the absence of illness, but by the presence of mental, spiritual, and emotional well-being and personal and cultural justice. Once you see yourself clearly and holistically in your mind's eye, then shift your attention to your journal. You will be more contemplative and ready to learn about yourself in a deeper, kinder, more empowering way.

When journaling, it can be especially important to write down negative thoughts because they are often automatic. Writing about them forces you to examine them, which can stop them from sabotaging you. Don't ruminate, but instead look for the lesson in whatever is on your mind or the blessing hidden within. Try to conclude each writing session with at least one positive thought that centers on gratitude. Centering on gratitude has been shown to be healing and motivating. As one of my yoga teachers taught me, "If you cannot be grateful for it, can you be grateful in it?"

PRACTICE

Take some time to breathe slowly and deeply for at least a minute, focusing on the sensations of your breath. Then, envision yourself, vibrant, strong and joyful. Use your journal to reflect on the following:

1. *What can you do to make journaling a habit?*
2. *What lessons have you learned that you are grateful for?*

Journal

Using the Five Whys and Motivational Interviewing to Create Change

Distant Memory

In Quality Improvement, we have a practice called the Five Whys, which is a methodology for root cause analysis.[3] It allows you to get below the surface and to dig down into the factors that created the problem. Let's combine this with considering the factors that motivate change, according to Motivational Interviewing, the technique extensive research shows can effectively inspire positive change. These motivating factors are best remembered with the mnemonic DANCRS: Desire, Ability, Need, Commitment, Reasons, and Steps already taken.[4]

PRACTICE

Take some time to breathe slowly and deeply for at least a minute, focusing on the sensations of your breath. Then, envision yourself vibrant, strong and joyful.

Recall a distant memory you have about food or body-image that somehow makes you feel bad. Use your journal to reflect on at least five of the following prompts:

1. *Why does this memory represent something about your desire for unconditional wellness?*
2. *Why does this memory represent something about your ability to unconditionally care for yourself?*

---

3   "5 Whys: Finding the Root Cause." Institute for Healthcare Improvement (IHI), 2020, http://www.ihi.org/resources/Pages/Tools/5-Whys-Finding-the-Root-Cause.aspx

4   R. Rhode. "Motivational Interviewing Review." *University of Arizona Center for Integrative Medicine*, Lecture, 2019

3. *Why does this memory represent what you feel you need to do to be truly well?*
4. *Why does this memory represent something about your commitment to unconditional wellness?*
5. *Why does this memory represent your reasons for promoting unconditional wellness?*
6. *Why does this memory represent the steps you have already taken on your path towards unconditional wellness?*

Journal

Now that you have spent some time focusing on the distant past, reflect on whether you should spend some more time there. This could be particularly valuable if your childhood or teen years included a lot of negative experiences involving food, body image, or exercise. If so, spend some more time reflecting on other distant memories. You need not choose the most painful memories, but try to reflect on something that evoked a sting. These stings we accumulate imprint themselves upon our spirits and our ways of subsequently treating ourselves. Only by delving into them can we understand ourselves and our own unique why.

Maybe go farther back in time, or to a more vibrant memory. Call to mind memories associated with multiple people in your life: both parents, older siblings, grandparents, people you dated, whomever feels relevant to you. Consider different phases of life: elementary school, junior high, high school, college, early work years, engagement, marriage, or the birth of a child.

There is no perfect way to do this reflection. Just do it. Whatever feels relevant will help you gain insight and self-awareness. Continuing repeating the exercise above until you feel finished, at least for now. Perhaps you will do this daily or every other day. The best way to learn from your past is to look at it differently, and this way of unearthing your own motivations is best done often enough that it becomes habitual. In this way, self-reflection and self-awareness can become habitual, just the way that self-criticism is already the default mode for many of us. Over time, this can change your own internal narrative about who you are and change your mindset to one centered on unconditional self-love.

Please do this from the perspective of thinking about how to make the best of your painful experiences and how to capitalize on your strengths. You may be tempted to place blame on others or yourself. Instead, think of how you can take back ownership of your body image. Start to let go of negative thoughts and cultivate growth. It is likely very hard to do this. Decompress afterwards with a loved one, or consider contacting a therapist.

PRACTICE

Take some time to breathe slowly and deeply for at least a minute, focusing on the sensations of your breath. Then, envision yourself: vibrant, strong, and joyful. Use your journal to reflect on the following prompts:

1. *Family History*
    a. Did your parents diet?
    b. Were they active?
    c. What was considered good food? Bad food?
    d. What health behaviors were rewarded? What were punished?
    e. What kind of messages were there regarding gender, health, and fitness?
    f. How were people viewed who were thin or lost weight? Why?
    g. How were people viewed that were obese? Why?
    h. How did your parents nourish themselves? How did they show love to you and your body?

Journal

2. *Your History*
    a. Make a photo scrapbook. In which photos did you *feel* your best? Look your best? What was the difference? When did you look your worst? Feel your worst? What was the difference?
    b. Make a timeline of your fitness. When did you feel your strongest and most powerful? Why? When did you feel your weakest and least vibrant? Why?
    c. If you are struggling with maintaining a healthy weight, when did it start, and what do you think are some factors?
    d. If you are struggling with disordered eating, when did it start, and what do you think were some factors?
    e. What do you need to relinquish in order to treat yourself well?

Journal

Recent Memory

Now that you have spent some time in the more distant past, consider a more recent memory, something in the last few days or weeks that is related to food, body image, or your beliefs about exercise.

PRACTICE

Take some time to breathe slowly and deeply for at least a minute, focusing on the sensations of your breath. Then, envision yourself vibrant, strong, and joyful. Use your journal to reflect on at least five of the following prompts:

1. *Why does this recent memory represent something about your desire for unconditional wellness?*
2. *Why does this recent memory represent something about your ability to unconditionally care for yourself?*
3. *Why does this recent memory represent what you feel you need to do to be truly well?*
4. *Why does this recent memory represent something about your commitment to unconditional wellness?*
5. *Why does this recent memory represent your reasons for promoting unconditional wellness?*
6. *Why does this recent memory represent the steps you have already taken on your path towards unconditional wellness?*

Journal

Notice what came up and how it might be connected to one of the more distant memories you wrote about. Is there a pattern, a tie, or an opposite? If you wrote about food, maybe write about another recent memory more directly connected to body image, or vice versa. If you wrote about exercise, maybe instead write now about inactivity. Switch it up. See what else is there. Do a little sleuthing into your own memories. Do you have a tendency, like many of us, to focus on what reinforces what you already believe? Do you tend to ignore or forget about experiences that maybe represent the opposite, or question your own strong beliefs about yourself and your own life? Pause here. Re-read the questions above and maybe write about this tendency if it is there. Let it flow.

Journal

PRACTICE

Take some time to breathe slowly and deeply for at least a minute, focusing on the sensations of your breath. Then, envision yourself vibrant, strong, and joyful. Use your journal to reflect on the following:

1. *Who are you with? Are you alone, with friends or family, a pet, or co-workers?*
2. *What are you doing while in this vibrant state? What are you not doing?*
3. *When is it? Time of day, season, phase of life.*
4. *Where are you? Outside, inside, at work, home, where you live now, versus somewhere else.*
5. *Why can you tell you are so unconditionally well in body, mind, and spirit?*

Journal

Notice what surprises you. What was different than the future you generally expect for yourself? Did you uncover a new possibility that you do not ordinarily allow yourself to daydream about? What might be indeed more positive, more vibrant, than the messages you, your family, or society, seem to tell you about what can be ahead?

Why Is Un-Less for You?

The fantastic thing about Un-Less is that it is suitable for everyone: someone wrestling with poor body image and self-care, obesity, anorexia, or bulimia. The focus is on becoming healthy inside and out.

Read below and see which unhealthy patterns, A through M, seem the most like yours and how the approach can help. Consider all of them, because few people fit into only one category. Circle all the letters you identify with.

Unhealthy Patterns

A   *"I tend to overeat, and I eat a lot of junk food. I have never been a healthy eater, and my family wasn't either. I have dieted before, but never consistently. I'm not accustomed to eating many fruits and veggies. I love fatty foods, and I have dessert with almost every meal. I feel like I need to change everything to get healthy, and it's overwhelming. Diets make me feel like I'm depriving myself, so I get miserable and give up quickly."* A This type of "all or nothing" mentality tends to center on eating what is familiar and comfortable. The great thing about Un-Less is that it doesn't recommend eliminating any food. It encourages you to choose the foods you do enjoy that energize and provide health benefits. As you learn more about the differences between physiologic and emotional hunger, you will give yourself more, not less, of the things your body truly desires. This will diminish the mindset that a diet is the answer. This, in turn, creates sustainable, long-term change and unconditional wellness.

B   *"I tend to eat healthy food, but I eat more than I should. I don't mind exercise, and I used to be athletic. However, I am discouraged now because I'm out of shape, don't have time, and overall just haven't made it a priority."* B This pattern is often indicative of people who have trouble being satisfied with moderation. You like to eat healthy foods, but your love of food makes it hard for you to stop yourself from having seconds and thirds. You like to exercise, but it seems like a waste to go for a half an hour power walk instead of the runs you used to do. In Un-Less, you will learn "moderation in all things but love," and you may find yourself enjoying your food more, as you learn to savor it. Also, you will find small bursts of exercises are easy enough to fit into your schedule, and that when you do, you may find it so rewarding you will make more time for it.

C   *"I tend to eat healthy when I feel good, but when I am anxious, bored, lonely, or have other unpleasant feelings, I tend to eat for comfort. I then feel guilty about it and try to compensate by eating very little afterwards, but I always end up soothing myself with food again, because I get so hungry, and feel so rotten."* C This type of emotional eating tends to happen to those who were soothed or bribed with food as children. You learned that a cupcake was a way to make things right, and you tend to reach for indulgences when things feel wrong. In addition, you desperately want to be healthy, so once you eat poorly, you beat yourself up for it. You then try to be overly restrictive, which just ends up making you miserable, and then you reach for a treat again. Although you may be of normal weight, your intake of nutritious foods is low. In Un-Less, you will learn to dine, not just eat. By eating for energy, you will feel vibrant, stabilizing your moods and learning new ways to self soothe that are not food-related. In this way, you will break your cycle, which is very much like a binge and purge cycle, though less extreme.

D "*I know a lot about nutrition, but I am so busy I never have the time to cook healthy meals or have healthy snacks. I end up overeating whatever is in front of me, and then I rush through it because I am famished.*" D You have a good grasp of what healthy eating habits are, but you have not made them a priority. With Un-Less, you will learn the necessity and value of prioritizing your own needs. This will allow you to be calmer and more efficient, which will make your hectic life easier. The Tips for Being Healthy on the Go will help you learn to find healthy snacks and meals everywhere, even the vending machine and the gas station. Also, journaling about your present circumstances and future goals will help you prioritize, freeing up time for healthier habits.

E "*I love food, cooking, and drinking. There is nothing more relaxing and fun for me than getting together with friends and sharing a fantastic meal. The only problem is, I do this too often, and I have put on weight over the years. I also tend to celebrate small victories, like finishing an assignment, with a treat, even when I'm not hungry.*" E You are a great lover of relaxation and "*la buena vida.*" However, your "here and now" focus has become baggage because you have become saddled with extra weight. Un-Less will help you find other ways of celebrating life and will help you make better choices about how to indulge. You will learn to tune into your body and to eat when you are hungry, not when you seek pleasure. Also, you may find that by listening to your body about food, and not your mind or heart, you will find that you actually crave healthy foods, not the indulgent things you think of as treats. By becoming more thoughtful about what you put in your body, you will learn to celebrate your own wellness, and that this is a gift you can give yourself every moment. You will find that a dinner out with friends is just as fun with healthy food. Also, even more encouraging, you won't have the "food hangover" the next day or feel guilty about overeating.

F *"I don't know why I'm overweight. I don't eat as much as other people, even thin people. I eat what I want to, but it's not exactly what you'd call a balanced diet. I guess I have a slow metabolism."* F As someone who is overweight but eats little, you may find that you feel better emotionally and physically by not trying to restrict your intake, since you are already good at limiting portion size. Un-Less will teach you about healthy eating behaviors and about eating for energy. Very likely, you will find you can lose weight while eating more often and a larger volume. When establishing your health baseline, your medical provider may also recommend some testing to rule out hormonal imbalances that could be contributing, as well.

G *"I am at a normal weight, but I know I'm not a healthy eater. I watch my portion sizes, but I tend to make poor choices in terms of nutrition. My body image is pretty realistic and healthy, but I know that I could benefit from becoming more positive."* G When you are at a normal weight, you may find little impetus to improve your eating habits, since so much of the focus on being healthy in our culture centers around being thin. However, choosing more nutritious foods can drastically improve your mood and energy. You will feel more vitality and look more vibrant. You will also pave the path for a healthy future. Establishing healthy eating habits will sustain you for the decades to come, when your body naturally loses lean muscle mass. Overall, Un-Less will help you most by increasing your mindfulness and self-understanding. You will also have the tools to be more loving to yourself and, therefore, increase your happiness.

H *"I wake up every morning determined to eat well. I am very careful about what I eat all day long, and people even comment that I always seem to be on a diet. I wish this were true. At night, when no one is paying attention, I let my guard down and indulge in all the things I avoided all day. I know this pattern makes no sense, so I try again almost every morning. I don't know why I binge at night, but it feels like an awful roller coaster ride. I want to take good care of myself. It's like I lose all control once I get home at the end of the day."* H This pattern is extremely common among obese people and even has a name, Night Eating Syndrome. For those who are motivated to be healthy, the public display of effort, eating healthy while around others, may feel imperative. However, at night, or in private, bingeing occurs, bringing an onslaught of guilt. This pattern is very difficult to break without deep introspection, which Un-Less can guide you through. You are not alone.

I *"I get so frustrated with my eating. I am hungry all the time. Or, at least, I think I am. I don't know. Maybe I just don't eat enough during my main meals, but I just don't feel good eating that much at any one time. I graze. To me, that feels better, because I never eat too much, which would stress me out. The problem is, I think I may eat too much overall because I am somewhat overweight. The whole thing just doesn't feel fair."* I This pattern is a confusing one to manage because there are conflicting schools of thought about how often people should eat. Many experts recommend mini-meals throughout the day to limit portion size, while others suggest that intermittent periods of fasting better regulate blood sugar hormones and decrease cellular aging. With Un-Less, you can shed this conflicting advice because you learn to tune into your own internal physiologic hunger cues and how to eat for real satiety. You will eat enough to feel powerful over time, developing your own natural reflective pattern.

J *"I am a healthy eater most of the time, but I drink or use marijuana frequently, and, when I'm intoxicated, I let my guard down and overindulge. I end up taking in a ton of calories from booze and the things I eat while partying."* J This pattern—healthy eating when you are sober and overindulging when you're partying—may be indicative of having trouble feeling comfortable and accepting yourself. When you're intoxicated, you let yourself give into the impulses that you feel all the time but usually keep in check. When you're drinking, however, you feel as though you have the freedom to do whatever you want. However, in the morning, you are hungover, not only from the alcohol, but from the guilt of overeating. With Un-Less, you will learn that food is not an enemy against which you need to be vigilant. By being less restrictive when you're sober, you will have less need to escape when you drink or use cannabis. By learning to be loving and accepting of yourself, you will be less inclined to go to extremes. On the whole, however, I suggest you discuss your use of substances with a medical or mental health professional if you have continued to use despite professional or personal problems. Un-Less can help you learn more about yourself through journaling and improve your body-image and eating habits, but it should be an adjunct to any additional support and treatment you may need.

K   *"I am able to stay at a reasonable weight, despite poor eating, because I exercise a ton. It's a terrible game of catch up. I know I will gain weight overtime if I keep eating like this, and the intense exercise is hard on my body."* K The constant cycle of overindulging in food and then trying to make up for it with intense exercise is a pattern that paves a slippery slope towards *exercise bulimia*. If you find yourself bingeing (eating compulsively and taking in a large number of calories in a short amount of time) and then pushing yourself physically, despite fatigue, dizziness, injury, or other symptoms, please consult a medical or mental health practitioner. Un-Less can help you learn more about yourself through journaling and improve your body image and eating habits, but it should be an adjunct to other treatment that you may need. On the other hand, if you do not have such an intense problem but feel as if you must carefully work off all the calories you take in, Un-Less can help you adopt a more loving pattern so your self-love is unconditional.

L   *"I'm at a fairly normal weight, but no matter what I do, I never feel thin enough. Sometimes I binge and then purge (throw up), make myself exercise for many hours, or take laxatives to get rid of the excess calories."* L This binge-and-purge cycle is indicative of *bulimia nervosa* and requires personalized support. Un-Less can help you learn more about yourself through journaling and may improve your body image and eating habits, but it should be an adjunct to other treatment. Please seek help from a medical or mental health professional to get expert support. When reading Un-Less, focus on the sections on self-exploration and learning to love yourself.

M *"I am at a normal weight, or underweight, though I never feel thin or fit enough. I find it hard to eat the way other people do because I am scared I will lose control and gain weight. This fear has taken over my life. I have stopped doing many things I love because my life is focused on controlling my eating and ensuring I exercise."* M This intense focus on weight and exercise is likely indicative of *anorexia nervosa*, and requires personalized support. Anorexia is treatable, but it is one of the deadliest mental health conditions. Please seek help now from a medical or mental health professional to get expert support. Un-Less can help you learn more about yourself through journaling and may help you improve your body image, but it should be adjunct to other critical treatment. When reading Un-Less, focus on the chapters on self-exploration and learning to love yourself.

PRACTICE

Take some time to breathe slowly and deeply for at least a minute, focusing on the sensations of your breath. Then, envision yourself vibrant, strong, and joyful. Use your journal to reflect on the following:

1. *What pattern(s) above fit you best?*
2. *Why?*
3. *Why not?*

Journal

The Un-Less Pledge

Below you will find a mantra and pledge that reviews Un-Less in its essence. The prayer and mantra are shortened versions of the pledge. Like any mantra, which means "mind tool," it can be useful to repeat to yourself, to center and relieve stress, in prayer or meditation. Speak them both aloud to yourself now and any time you need encouragement. Use them like many people use the Serenity Prayer, a poem used in many settings, such as Alcoholics Anonymous, to center and provide strength.

Serenity Prayer

Grant me the serenity to accept the things I cannot change, the courage to change the things I can, and the wisdom to know the difference.

The Un-Less Pledge

I am a beautiful person right now. There may be ugliness in my past, but it was not because I was too skinny or too heavy. It was because I did not treat myself in a loving way. By learning about why I made the choices I did, I can leave them behind. By examining my history, I will decide upon my future. I will help my body thrive by being mindful. I will be present and think about the effects of my choices. I used to make my body struggle. Now, I choose to nourish myself.

I am not giving myself rules against which I might rebel. I am giving myself principles, so I will be a principled, mindful person. When I am hungry, I will dine on food that nourishes me. I will therefore feel satiated, focused, energized, and peaceful. I will be active so that my muscles grow strong and I feel powerful. I will challenge my body, but I will not push it too hard. I will let it rest. I will sleep as much as I need to wake up alert and motivated.

Lastly, I will have a sense of humor and remember that health begins with heal. I will not take myself too seriously, and I will remember that I don't have to be perfect. Good enough is good enough. I am healing myself because I deserve more, not less. I am lovely. I love me, unconditionally, now.

The Un-Less Prayer

I choose to nourish myself through my principles and actions. Health begins with heal. I am healing myself because I deserve more, not less. I am lovely. I love me, unconditionally, now.

The Un-Less Mantra

Unconditional Love

Try matching "unconditional" with your inhale, and "love" with your exhale for a simple concentrative meditation.

PRACTICE

Take some time to breathe slowly and deeply for at least a minute, focusing on the sensations of your breath. Then, envision yourself vibrant, strong, and joyful. Use your journal to reflect on the following:

1. *How did it feel to say the prayer and mantra aloud?*
2. *What else can you repeat to yourself for grounding?*

Journal

Maybe make a few copies of the mantra or key words on sticky notes, and post them all over. Put them anywhere you know might trigger you, or anywhere you may need to be reminded that you are wonderful just as you are and you deserve loving-kindness and unconditional wellness.

PRACTICE

Take the time to write out the prayer and mantra above in your own handwriting. Remember, motivational interviewing shows us that we believe what we ourselves say, so take the time to recite and write these words. Only then will they become powerful tools for transformation.

Journal

PART II

Philosophical Principles

Now that you have taken the time to consider the messages, both explicit and implicit, that you have inherited from your family and community, you can decide what you what to carry forward and what to leave behind. The following bedrock principles of Un-Less can give you guidance for re-framing the messages you have received and will improve your relationship with food and body-image. They are all equally important and are all key to healing.

Health Begins with Heal

One key reason people do not care for themselves well is due to trauma or loss. In a mild form, it is why we classically binge on ice cream during a break-up. However, it can have much more serious consequences, as well. For example, the Adverse Childhood Experiences study of over 15,000 people revolutionized our understanding of the impact of abuse and how it can relate to weight. Many obese women with a history of sexual or physical abuse felt little motivation to lose weight. They explained that the excess fat felt like a safety blanket, fending off unwanted attention.

Therefore, it is especially critical to deeply consider the reasons we make poor choices, because every reason makes some sense. If it did not, we would not repeat that action enough to create an unhealthy habit. Actions are not unhealthy; habits and patterns can be. One bowl of ice cream is not unhealthy; a tub each evening is. Eating salad for dinner is healthy; making yourself eat it every night is not.

If this process of soul searching brings up a history of trauma or abuse, reach out to someone who can help. Just as I benefitted from therapy, so too would almost everyone else. You will not need it forever, but having a knowledgeable, caring person who listens and whom you don't have to care for can be liberating and provide incomparable breakthroughs. Don't be too proud to open up. Even "normal" losses and transitions, such as grief, divorce, and becoming a parent, are profound life changes that can rock you. Learning how to best soothe yourself during these times can make them into growth experiences, paving the way for joy and appreciation for new opportunities.

Our mental and emotional health determines our physical well-being. Your wellness is a priority. Taking action to care for yourself is responsible. It is the best gift you can give yourself and those you love. Health begins with heal.

PRACTICE

Take some time to breathe slowly and deeply for at least a minute, focusing on the sensations of your breath. Then, envision yourself vibrant, strong, and joyful. Use your journal to reflect on the following:

1. *What is a trauma or loss you have had that makes it hard to make healthy choices?*
2. *What kinds of things can you do to help yourself heal?*

Journal

Reasoned, Not Rigid

Imagine a thick, dense tree trunk. It seems so strong. However, it cannot bend. It fractures in a hurricane, compared to thin bendable branches that can react to the flow. Being dense and rigid, therefore, creates tension and weakness. You, too, will break from rigidity, which is why Un-Less does not give you rules to abide by. Rules create rigidity and compel us to follow something outside of ourselves, which usually makes us feel inadequate, breaking us down emotionally. Rules also make us to want to rebel, to break free. Rules are the hallmark of diets, so the avoidance of rules underlines that Un-Less is intentionally not a diet.

So, what then will guide you, if not rules and rigidity? Reason. Reason is the interplay between logic (the intellect) and emotion (the intuition). You will use mindfulness to build your depth of reasoning so you are not following rules but making choices. You will not say, "I cannot have cake," but you will instead ask yourself, "Is this the time I will have cake?" There is no need to rebel from your well-reasoned self.

Reasoning, therefore, builds strength, decreases tension, and increases flexibility. It also creates lightness rather than density, clarity rather than opacity. This keeps your choices exciting and empowering. It is yoga of the mind.

PRACTICE

Take some time to breathe slowly and deeply for at least a minute, focusing on the sensations of your breath. Then, envision yourself vibrant, strong, and joyful. Use your journal to reflect on the following:

1. *How has being rigid undermined your strength in the past?*
2. *In what ways do you want to become more flexible?*

Journal

Soothe

The journaling of Un-Less helps you delve into the emotional triggers that have led to poor self-care. Many times, this will mean taking a close look at how you were raised or how your relationships may be causing you harm, and it will hurt. Do not crack open the cookie drawer, a beer, or force yourself to run 10 miles. Crack open your journal, call a friend, or do some other relaxing activity. This process is about learning to soothe yourself in ways that do not involve eating, or even exercise. You may find a bath, pedicure, watching football, or even masturbating are all great ways to change your outlook towards the positive.

Vibrant health begins with doing things for the right reasons, and emotions can lead us far off track if we are not tuned into how they are influencing action. One framework for tuning into oneself is the HALT system. HALT stands for Hungry, Angry, Lonely, and Tired. It was originally conceptualized by Alcoholics Anonymous as a way of noting when people are vulnerable to relapse from substance abuse. It can help you identify the best way to soothe yourself. If you are truly hungry, then please, by all means, nourish yourself. But if you are angry, lonely, or tired, those chips, or even carrots, are not going to help one bit. Target your self-care to what you need.

Anger, in particular, is destructive. Don't let frustration with others lead you to take poor care of yourself. Deal with your anger constructively. Explain why you are feeling as you are, using "I" statements to avoid adding fuel to the fire. For example, say, "I feel hurt when you don't tell me you are going to be home late," not "When you are late it is rude!" Ask for an apology, and then accept it. Or, perhaps you are just angry with yourself? These things are complicated. That is why your journal is there. Pick it up.

Loneliness is a state which also has profound effects on self-care. When we feel lonely, many of us often over-indulge, free from the sense that others may judge. This is an undercurrent of the sentiment in HALT: be cautious that when you are feeling lonely, you may go overboard. Conversely, some people do not let themselves relax and enjoy when they are alone. As an example, let me share an experience I had. I was travelling alone for a conference. After a lovely dinner out on my own, on a gorgeous plaza in Valencia, the waiter asked me, "I hope you don't mind, but what is a lovely person like you doing eating alone?" He meant it as kindly as possible and was truly inquisitive. But under the current of compassion, I felt a tension. Why should I not have a lovely dinner by myself? Why hole up in my hotel room just because no one else could join me? I am sure he meant to suggest it was someone else's loss, but we must be careful not to absorb the idea that food, as pleasure, is something people should only enjoy with others. I have a friend who shared with me that she used to skip dinner when she was alone because she felt as though she didn't really deserve a proper meal if it wasn't with others. This is not to say that loneliness is foolish. It is good to crave the company of those you care about. My dinner in Valencia would indeed have been better if I had someone to laugh with about my adventures or simply to savor the cuisine with. However, life comes with social times and solitary ones. Make sure you nourish yourself all the time, in balance, so you can enjoy the blessings of each.

Lastly, HALT reminds us that being tired, or fatigued, is also a state which limits good decision-making. Making sure you get enough sleep and eat for energy is key. Similarly, making sure you have enough emotional reserve is just as important. Remember, the glass is not half full or half empty; it is refillable. You can replenish yourself.

Soothing is a central principle of Un-Less because poor health is more about poor self-nurturing than it is about nutrition or lack of activity. Indeed, someone who has some poor health behaviors can actually be surprisingly healthy. My grandfather, for example, did many things "wrong" in terms of health. He smoked a pipe, ate without concern for nutrition, enjoyed his Old Fashioned every night, and did not exercise. However, he was vibrant and sharp into his mid-90s because he never overdid any of those things. He also had many healthy ways to soothe himself. He had positive relationships, hobbies, and meaningful work, which kept him mentally active and inspired.

When we consider ourselves as beings that indeed need fuel but also need so many other sources of nourishment to flourish, it becomes a lot less critical to do every little thing "right." That is why Un-Less does not offer you an exact formula for wellness. Instead, learning how to soothe yourself in healthy ways, to combat the daily barrage of stress, is what will ultimately lead to *your* best life.

Indeed, Western science is now recognizing what Eastern practitioners have been explaining for centuries: that stress is a major factor in most illnesses. Extensive research is now showing that stress, poor nutrition, and inactivity cause inflammation, which triggers numerous disease processes, including cancers, heart disease, and many others. Wellness really is the integration of mind, body, and spirit, emotionally and biochemically.

While we cannot remove stress as a whole in our lives (nor should we: it is one way for guiding us towards what is good) we must take action to decrease its effects. Thankfully, eating well and being mindful and active counteract this stress-inflammation cascade. So, you are on your way. Journaling will also tune you in to what changes you need to decrease your own stress, from work, relationships, etc.

As you learn what you need to do to soothe yourself, you are literally healing yourself, inside and out.

PRACTICE

Take some time to breathe slowly and deeply for at least a minute, focusing on the sensations of your breath. Then, envision yourself vibrant, strong, and joyful. Use your journal to reflect on the following:

1. *How have you used anger against yourself in the past?*
2. *How might you soothe yourself differently in the future?*

Journal

Radiant, Not Clean

One popular word in the wellness industry is "clean." It may be used to mean the opposite of processed, or free from artificial additives. It can also refer to going on a "cleanse," which can vary from fasting, to restricting specific foods, to taking in only fruits and veggies, to, well, literally anything. The web offers endless ideas, ranging from reasonable to dangerous.

I advise against typical cleanses for multiple reasons. First, they are generally very restrictive, and therefore unsustainable, so there is no long-term benefit. In addition, even healthy things like natural juice are not meant to be enjoyed in isolation. A good thing can quickly go from a healthy choice to an unbalanced practice, even triggering dangerous electrolyte imbalances and nutrient deficiencies. Nevertheless, even for people who do not use the term in an extreme manner, I still suggest we abandon "clean." Why? Because the opposite is "dirty."

To think of ourselves as dirty is to immediately invoke spiritual and sexual connotations of either guilt or indecency. It immediately reinforces the notion that we need to be pure to be good. The pursuit of purity has been plaguing people for eons. It pushes us away from listening to our own instincts and leads us to believe we are not good if we don't ascribe to a set of rules. In Un-Less, healthy eating is about embracing our wants and needs and pleasure. It embraces foods that are natural, but also provides plenty of wiggle-room for the "naughtier" delights of life: treats and delicacies, or a night on the couch with Netflix.

We do not need others to tell us that what is clean is good and what is dirty is bad. We can learn to listen to our own intuition. When we do so mindfully, we will find that our bodies generally want what is healthy. That is why they feel awful when we fill them will crap and allow them to get weak! We can trust our bodies to guide us how to feel good, as long as we stop telling them they are bad. What we should cleanse is our hearts, letting go of guilt. Guilt only does one thing to health, and that is undermine it. As soon as we have guilt, we have rebellion, and, when we rebel against ourselves, we are the losers.

So, if we are not trying to clean, what are we to do? How about we attempt to radiate? Radiate energy? Joy? Warmth? All of these are images of emission, giving off power. In Un-Less, you are not seeking to establish control (remember, "reasoned, not rigid"). Instead, your goal is to share your light, which is to empower yourself and others. When we eat foods that are energizing and make us feel powerful, we are eating radiantly. When we care for ourselves, be it through movement, meditation, pampering, or simply laughing, we are recharging our batteries. Think of yourself as a source of radiance, and it will be much simpler to know what will give you the power to feel your best.

PRACTICE

Take some time to breathe slowly and deeply for at least a minute, focusing on the sensations of your breath. Then, envision yourself vibrant, strong, and joyful. Use your journal to reflect on the following:

1. *What would it mean to you to let go of the notion that healthy means clean?*
2. *What practices make you feel radiant?*

Journal

Sweetness

Sweetness is a lot more than a flavor. It is the essence of cheer and warmth. We all need sweetness in our lives. Perhaps there really is a reason that dessert is "stressed" spelled backward! Indeed, although there is absolutely room in any healthy eating approach for dessert, oftentimes, when we are craving chocolate, what we really need is emotional sweetness: a hug, some tenderness, to feel beloved.

Many people take poor care of themselves because others have taken poor care of them. They end up continuing the same pattern, reinforcing what they were shown. If you have a history of abuse, neglect, or just a bad heartbreak, chances are you need some sweetness that cannot come from food. Again, the value of therapy cannot be understated.

PRACTICE

Take some time to breathe slowly and deeply for at least a minute, focusing on the sensations of your breath. Then, envision yourself vibrant, strong, and joyful. Use a piece of paper, not your journal, to reflect on the following:

1. Write down one thing that you are resentful of. Define this as anything you are "re-sending," perseverating about, or cannot let go of.
2. Then, let yourself write a stream of consciousness about all the reasons why you FEAR it. (FEAR here stands for False Evidence Appearing Real.)
3. End by shredding or burning your paper.

I learned this exercise from a yoga teacher who introduced it as a way for us to expel negative thoughts before meditation. You can do it anytime you find yourself getting anxious. It can be a great way to relieve stress and prepare yourself to let in the sweetness, be it in the form of a date, a long weekend with friends, or any source of joy. We need sweetness, and letting go of bitterness is the best way to taste it. So, whenever you are about to pick up a candy bar, ask yourself whether it is the sweetness you truly want. If it is, go for it, in a reasonable quantity, especially if it is high quality and will really feel special. If not, maybe find your dog, play fetch, and have a cuddle, and then see if you still need sweetness. Maybe not. Or maybe a perfect summer peach will be just what the NP ordered.

PRACTICE

Take some time to breathe slowly and deeply for at least a minute, focusing on the sensations of your breath. Then, envision yourself vibrant, strong, and joyful. Use your journal to reflect on the following:

1. *What kind of sweetness is missing from your life right now?*
2. *What can you do to change that?*

Journal

Spice

Similar to sweetness, we all need spice in our lives. If you are like my husband, you live for hot sauce and may even feel down without it. The capsaicin in peppers is a natural booster of serotonin (our main feel-good neurotransmitters), so there is some real science there. The spice I am focusing on here though is the "variety is the spice of life" type. Indeed, a mundane routine will kill motivation, stifle creativity, and bring you down. Seek out new experiences, try new foods, activities, and sources of entertainment. Very often, we make poor choices because we have little excitement in our lives and we want distraction or stimulation. Create room in your life for newness, and the lure of the couch won't seem so strong. When you are stuck in a rut (professionally, in relationships, or otherwise), food or exercise may be the first thing you seek to feel a sense of adventure.

While it can be great to try new cuisines or go for a run, first examine your day and think more critically about why you feel a need to escape. Your journal is a great place for you to identify these patterns. Adding a section about what you were thinking about right before any episodes of poor eating may cue you into what is pushing you towards escapism. I know whenever I am inspired in my work and relationships, taking care of myself comes naturally. Perhaps it's because I am getting input telling me I am valued, and therefore it makes it easier for me to value myself. However, when I felt less satisfied and stuck, it is much more likely for me to act in self-defeating ways. This drama is not the kind of useful spice that drives enthusiasm for change! So, shake things up in your life to make your world just as fresh as your intake.

PRACTICE

Take some time to breathe slowly and deeply for at least a minute, focusing on the sensations of your breath. Then, envision yourself vibrant, strong, and joyful. Use your journal to reflect on the following:

1. *What part of your life feels dull and needs a little shaking up?*
2. *What can you do to try something new?*

Journal

Mindful Dining

Chances are you conceptualize dining as something that includes white tablecloths and candles. You are not wrong. It is the act of eating which is greater than just eating; it incorporates the surrounding sights, sounds, smells, social culture, and overall ambience. And, it is not reserved for restaurants.

Most books on health focus on food and eating. Food is generally labeled bad or good, and healthy eating is seen as simply an act to relieve hunger and provide nutrients. However, this is a recipe for misery. No actions are truly bad; only patterns are. The same is true with food. Just as food is fuel, so, too, we are not robots, and we should not eat for fuel only. While we should consider the nutritional content of our choices, we should be eating to dine, not eating to fuel. Why? Simply because life is meant to be loved, not worked through! Mindful eating, therefore, becomes mindful dining.

Pay attention to taste, color, texture, and smell. These all increase your sensory experience and your pleasure; they don't depend on how much you eat! This is holistic, mindful dining. Use your eyes, ears, nose, and mouth. Chew, really chew. Tune into the sensation and one small serving of ice cream can become plenty.

Anytime you can make eating more pleasant, do so. Set the table. Light candles. Play music. You would do these things for guests. Why not for yourself? If you're not at home, do whatever else you can to focus on your food. Pull the car to the side of the road. Eat your bag lunch on a bench in the park instead of at your desk. Make your meal an experience. Put away your phone; turn off the TV.

Eating is one of great sensory experiences of life, and it is a social activity that brings people together. It is meant to be pleasure-filled, not to bring you stress. Whenever possible, dine with those you care about, and share your healthy recipes and food with them. Unconditional wellness becomes a lot easier when those around you are on board as well.

PRACTICE

Take some time to breathe slowly and deeply for at least a minute, focusing on the sensations of your breath. Then, envision yourself vibrant, strong, and joyful. Use your journal to reflect on the following:

1. *What elements of ambience can you enhance at home to make eating more like dining?*
2. *What about at your office or other places you often eat?*

Journal

Savor

Just as we should dine, not eat, so, too, should we do all we can to savor our food. To savor is to slow down and tune into all the sensations the food offers: the smell, taste, color, texture. You love to eat, so why not slow down? You'll get to eat for twice as long! And, it will be easier to tell when you're full, since your stomach's appetite signals don't communicate satiety to the brain for at least twenty minutes. Interestingly, even healthy foods trigger a surge of stress hormones when eaten too fast.[5]

If you struggle with speed, you may find it helpful to eat with chopsticks or a smaller spoon. You may also find eating with others slows you down, since you talk. It tends to make the whole experience feel more like dining, as well. If small talk feels painful, remember, someone is only a stranger once. Who knows? You may make a break-through connection or simply a new friend.

PRACTICE

Take some time to breathe slowly and deeply for at least a minute, focusing on the sensations of your breath. Then, envision yourself vibrant, strong, and joyful. Use your journal to reflect on the following:

1. *What helps you slow down when you are eating?*
2. *How can you better organize your day to feel less rushed at each meal?*

5   R. Bonakdar. "Integrative Management of Metabolic Pain and Headache: Focus on Nutritional Strategies." *University of Arizona Center for Integrative Medicine*, Lecture, 2019

Journal

Hunger

One primary reason people don't stick to healthy eating is physical hunger. It is usually because they may have eaten too little previously, waited too long before eating again, or ate something that created a blood sugar dip and led to hunger earlier than anticipated. Un-Less includes strategies for all of these issues.

Hunger is not the enemy, though. It is a natural and desirable process that lets you listen to your body regarding when it needs energy. The key to preventing poor choices is learning to tune into your hunger and to eat when you are appropriately hungry.

Start by considering whether you have true physiologic hunger, which grows slowly over time, is felt in the abdomen, and can be decreased by consuming any food group. Emotional hunger, on the other hand, tends to come on quickly. It gets triggered by an experience. It seems to reside in the head or heart and is accompanied by longing for a particular food-type. There are no real physical symptoms because it is not true hunger, but you may have symptoms of anxiety, such as nausea, or palpitations.

Once you determine if you are physiologically hungry, rank your hunger from zero to three: zero is not at all hungry, one is somewhat hungry, two is moderately hungry, and three is ravenous. The goal is to eat when you feel a one or two. Waiting until you are a three is setting yourself up for making poor choices. It is also uncomfortable, which is your body's way of telling you it is not healthy. It is not healthy to wait until you are nauseated, shaky, irritable, dizzy, or having difficulty concentrating. You should feel good when you eat! When you learn to listen to your body and eat when your body needs energy, you will be eating for wellness. Sometimes you will end up at a three because you were super busy or ate something that did not sustain you long enough. Mindful journaling will help you look back on that and will lead you to insights on how to prevent it.

For many people who have not been listening to their body's signals regarding eating, tuning into hunger and letting it lead can be tough. This applies to those who have been eating due to boredom, temporal cues ("It's noon: time for lunch!"), sensation-seeking, or otherwise "comfort eating." In many ways, these signals constitute mental or emotional hunger and will not be truly satisfied by food. Conversely, this also applies to those who have been restricting themselves from eating, even when hungry. Lastly, some people take medications that affect hunger and satiety and make it hard to trust their own bodies. That is why you have your journal: to be mindful, reflective, and to chart your progress over time.

Also, though I advise you listen to your body, not a clock, it is wise to check in with yourself about every five to six hours. Many times, we are in mentally absorbing tasks and then finish and suddenly realize we are famished. Prevent this by keeping healthy snacks nearby and visible, if you have this tendency.

Remember, it is your responsibility, and yours alone, to give your body what it needs. It is not your partner's responsibility to make a meal at exactly a certain time. You do not have license to be a jerk just because you let yourself get to a three. I call this person "Hangry," and I have no patience when my husband turns into him! You do not get to unleash this demon on others (or yourself!) because you were unprepared. Take care of business.

PRACTICE

Take some time to breathe slowly and deeply for at least a minute, focusing on the sensations of your breath. Then, envision yourself vibrant, strong, and joyful. Use your journal to reflect on the following:

1. *What holds you back from following hunger cues?*
2. *How can you better pay attention to how HALT (Hunger, Anger, Loneliness, Tiredness) might be affecting your choices?*

Journal

Sustain

Another word for food is sustenance. Food's very job is to sustain us. However, as you know, there are many times you eat when you not sustained and instead are hungry a short while later. This happens for two primary reasons. You may not be choosing enough food or the right foods.

The first reason is clear: you don't eat enough, and you get hungry. That's actually okay. Again, hunger is not the enemy. It will take some time to learn how much food your body needs to stay satisfied for the normal periods between intakes.

Note, I did not say meals. I want you to get rid of the concept that you need to eat three meals and then, maybe, snacks. No. You need to learn to listen to your body and learn to respond to its cues. What defines a snack versus a meal anyway? You "get" to eat more? Nonsense: you should always eat as much as it takes to provide yourself with sustenance. Or are meals defined as such because they occur morning, midday, and evening? Again, nonsense. You should dine whenever makes sense based on your sleep schedule. Avoid eating heavily in the hours before bedtime to improve sleep and optimize blood sugar levels.

Sustenance is about more than the amount or timing of food. In actuality, it is about the balance and quality of food—the quality of energy that determines the type of power. You want to feel like a superhero? Don't gas up with "products" that won't give you super power. Nourishing yourself takes a lot more than just simply giving yourself food. You need sustenance, and sustenance is defined by quality foods, in the right balance, when you need the energy.

PRACTICE

Take some time to breathe slowly and deeply for at least a minute, focusing on the sensations of your breath. Then, envision yourself vibrant, strong, and joyful. Use your journal to reflect on the following:

1. *What kinds of foods sustain your energy the best?*
2. *What makes you feel powerful and radiant after you eat it?*

Journal

Satiety

Just as hunger is about more than how empty your stomach is, so, too, is satiety also more complex than how full you are. Indeed, satiety is more related to sustenance, to feeling satisfied. It is more conceptual than physical—that is why you may feel stuffed but still have "room for dessert." Learning how to feel satiated requires multiple elements of self-knowledge.

First, what do I really want? That does not mean what do you crave, but what do you, as a whole person, need right now? Again, it may be more emotional than physical, so consider this. If it is true physiologic hunger, think about what you have had already recently. Have you had a lot of veggies but no fruit? It would likely be good, then, to have fruit. Have you had lots of animal products but no plant sources of protein? It would likely be good, then, to have a meal centered on beans or legumes. Thinking this way will ensure balance and novelty.

From another perspective, healthy eating is also about helping yourself relax. Be mindful of which foods help you relax. Creamy foods? Salty? Sour? Once you notice this, it is easier to replace less healthy choices with better ones because you know it's a taste sensation you want, not a food.

This idea is very important because this is another way that Un-Less is different from a diet. Diets tell you eating for sensation is bad and sticking to rules is good. However, rules only create rebellion. If you are craving chips and are drawn to salt and crunch, but you eat yogurt instead because it seems healthier, you will often eat the yogurt, then something else "good," and then, eventually, (after you are definitely no longer hungry!) eat the chips. You end up overeating because you did not tune into what would really satisfy you. If, in the first place, you ate popcorn, a whole grain with lots of fiber, then your craving for salt and crunch would be satisfied in a healthier way.

In Un-Less, you are not trying to get rid of cravings. Instead, you are listening to your body. When you are hungry, you eat. You eat food that matches the sensation you want, while letting the principles of healthy eating guide your choices. Think of cravings not as bad things to be ignored, nor impulses to follow willy-nilly, but as a way for your body to tell you what it is drawn to and what will satisfy you. By taking the emphasis off saying "no" to food and onto listening to yourself, you show yourself respect and facilitate unconditional wellness.

The second aspect of self-knowledge required for achieving satiety is thinking about sustenance, namely, not just what do I want right now, but what will sustain me for my next activities. (Note that I wrote activities, not hours.) Are you going to be watching a movie? You don't need much power. Are you going to hike to the top of Yosemite Falls? You definitely need to give your body both short- and long-acting energy. Learning what kind of power you need will keep you feeling vibrant. In general, you will feel most even and satiated if you eat whole foods, always combining complex carbohydrates with protein and healthy fats to stabilize blood sugar.

The last element of self-knowledge is tuning into when you have had enough. One Japanese principle may be of use here. It is "Hara hachi bun me," roughly translated as "Eat until you are 80% full." It is an idea about far more to me than just calculating how full you are, which is quite difficult since stomachs stretch. Instead, it refers to taking all that you need and not more. As above, if you have just finished eating, it is likely you are fuller than your brain knows. Also, I take it to mean that you are leaving enough for others so everyone has what they need. We're all in this together! Lastly, it may promote longevity. Okinawans, who follow the principle, have one of the highest life expectancies on earth. One Japanese philosopher, Yasutani, advised his students to eat only eighty percent of their capacity, saying, "Eight parts of a full stomach sustain the man; the other two sustain the doctor."

From a practical standpoint, avoid bringing the serving bowl with you to the table or grazing in front of a buffet. Make your plate before you start your meal, and make it as full as you likely need to be satiated. Sit down and dine. Tune in and enjoy. If you still find it hard to determine when you are satisfied, use a scale similar to the one used to determine hunger. Consider from zero to three how satiated you are, and compare it perhaps to how hungry you still are. Are your feelings unsatisfied even though you are no longer hungry? You likely have mental or emotional needs to attend to. Distinguishing between physical and emotional hunger is a tricky challenge, but it is one that allows you to nourish yourself holistically and to promote loving-kindness and unconditional wellness.

PRACTICE

Take some time to breathe slowly and deeply for at least a minute, focusing on the sensations of your breath. Then, envision yourself vibrant, strong, and joyful. Use your journal to reflect on the following:

1. *What are some healthier alternatives to foods you often crave, which provide the same basic sensation (e.g. sweet for sweet, salty for salty)?*
2. *What delicious antioxidant-rich foods do you enjoy and leave you feeling satisfied?*

Journal

Nourish

By now, I hope you have noticed that I use the word nourish quite liberally. In Un-Less, it means far more than nutritious "nourishing food." Instead, it incorporates the mental and emotional. To nourish is to care for, to nurture. Therefore, it contains the tenderness that you are learning to give yourself. For example, an apple is a healthy food, but if it is all you allow yourself to eat for lunch, you are not nourishing yourself. You are not showing yourself love. You are not giving yourself enough to be well. This is similar to the difference between healthy food and healthy eating. Also, nourishing yourself encompasses far more than giving yourself fuel.

To nourish yourself, you must care for yourself as a whole person: body, mind, and spirit. First, in terms of body, you deserve everything an animal needs to thrive—nutrition, sunlight, movement, air. In terms of mind, you deserve to have stimulation, novelty, learning. Lastly, in terms of spirit, you deserve tenderness, excitement, purpose, inspiration. Un-Less calls upon you to give yourself all the things you would give someone you love.

This book will give you lots of suggestions on how to improve your eating and movement. Sunlight and air are pretty self-explanatory. Only you know, though, what will give you stimulation, novelty, learning, tenderness, and excitement. That is why you are keeping a journal that is about far more than food. You are an animal, not a robot, and an animal with a sophisticated consciousness that deserves a rich life that you love! Start examining what will nourish you as a whole person.

PRACTICE

Take some time to breathe slowly and deeply for at least a minute, focusing on the sensations of your breath. Then, envision yourself vibrant, strong, and joyful. Use your journal to reflect on the following:

1. *What is your favorite way to nourish your mind?*
2. *Your spirit?*
3. *Your body?*

Journal

Nature

A resounding premise of Un-Less is that nature is the source of wellness. Indeed, every time we human beings think we can create something better than nature, we fail. For example, baby formula is an adequate substitute that is sometimes required, but breastfeeding is better for both baby and mother. Hydrogenated (trans) fats are oils that scientists created as a way to extend the shelf-life of foods. They thought they could also help us avoid the cholesterol found in animal fats. However, decades of research have revealed that these unnatural compounds are far worse than the natural saturated fats in bacon and butter. In sum, we are much better off nourishing our bodies with substances found in nature and as close to their natural state as possible.

Un-Less encourages you to love food. Food is energy, and your body is an organism that needs high-quality energy. What's better quality, Cheetos or a peach? Ho Hos or almonds? Which will leave you full, satiated, energized, and focused?

In the words of esteemed health journalist Michael Pollan, healthy food boils down to the following: "Eat food. Mostly plants. Not too much." What does he mean by this "eat food?" Of course, you must eat food. What else is there? Alas, there is so much more. What Pollan means is that we should be eating as naturally as possible: things that grow, not things that are made. What grows? Vegetables and fruits, grains, beans, nuts, and animals: what everyone ate until about 100 years ago.

We are animals, and, as omnivores, we are meant to eat other animals and plants. (Do you want to be vegetarian or vegan? No problem. Just ensure you are getting all your required nutrients.) Look in your kitchen. Does the food look like actual animals or plants? Yes? Then chances are you have nutritious food, full of the compounds your body needs to thrive. No? Then the "food" you have is probably actually better termed a "product," something man-made that is edible.

This is not sophisticated science, and it is not meant to be. You don't need to know sophisticated science to eat well. For now, though, you just need to know that, generally, the closer something it is to its natural state, the better it is for you. And, until recently, that was just common sense.

I should mention the value of caring for nature as we care for ourselves. Indeed, buying organic food is better for our soil and water supply, and it is also better for our bodies. The added bonus is that organic foods are themselves more vibrant. Blueberries, for example, that are not sprayed with pesticides to protect them, create more natural compounds to protect themselves. These become fabulous antioxidants which decrease inflammation. So, when you buy organic blueberries, you are getting more blueberry! They may be more expensive, yes, but they are a better value. If cost is a major deterrent for you, avoid, at least, the produce with thin skins. These types, often called the Dirty Dozen, are those where the pesticides are most likely to leach into the parts you eat. Examples are berries, peaches, nectarines etc.

Lastly, we must consider that our entire bodies depend on vitamins and minerals to have optimal enzymatic functioning. When we do not eat in a way that includes diverse vegetables and fruits, we risk missing out on the optimal level of these vital nutrients. Indeed, since our soil is now becoming depleted throughout the world, our plants (and the animals who eat them) take in fewer vitamins and minerals from the soil. This can have devastating but subtle health consequences. For example, our bodies need B vitamins to convert tryptophan, an amino acid (from protein), into two key compounds: serotonin, the mood boosting neuro-transmitter, and melatonin, which promotes sleep. Researchers are finding that a sub-optimal intake (not frank deficiency, which is more rare) of B vitamins is therefore tied to low mood and poor recovery after trauma.[6] The good news is that supplementation of B vitamins after trauma also appears to reduce the length of time people experience it (i.e. reduces Post Traumatic Stress Disorder). So, our poor soil and a diet without sufficiently healthy plants may partially explain the mental illness and poor sleep that are becoming all too common in our world.

PRACTICE

Take some time to breathe slowly and deeply for at least a minute, focusing on the sensations of your breath. Then, envision yourself vibrant, strong, and joyful. Use your journal to reflect on the following:

1. *What excites you about eating a more natural diet?*
2. *What are your favorite whole and minimally-processed foods?*

---

6   B. Kaplan, "Nutrition Above the Neck." *University of Arizona Center for Integrative Medicine,* Lecture, 2019.

Journal

Color

Speaking of blueberries, color is another key consideration. Color is nature's most obvious way of giving us information about nutrition. If a food is colorful, it will make you feel vibrant, too! The compounds that make up the naturally-occurring colors of nature are robust antioxidants and provide other benefits, as well. Beta-carotene, for example, which gives beets their glorious purple color, is glorious for us as well. It is converted to Vitamin A in the liver, boosting eye health, skin, fertility, and immunity. Overall, when you fill your plate with colorful fruits and vegetables, you are giving yourself far more than fuel. You are making the meal more interesting and healthier. Consider your plate as a canvas. Paint yourself a meal of beauty, abundant with the natural colors of plants that are reflective of their antioxidant phytonutrients that prevent disease and reduce inflammation.[7]

Similarly, a lack of color shows a lack of these same beneficial compounds. White rice and white potatoes are less nutritious than their colorful counterparts. Seek out brown, purple, and orange versions. Try grains that include the husks, which maximize fiber and phytonutrients. Any food that starts off with color and then is bleached and processed to be "refined" has lost much of its natural value.

7   D. Minich. "The Science and Art of Creativity for Healing." *Academy of Integrative Health and Medicine Conference*, Lecture, 2019.

PRACTICE

Take some time to breathe slowly and deeply for at least a minute, focusing on the sensations of your breath. Then, envision yourself vibrant, strong, and joyful. Use your journal to reflect on the following:

1. *What are your favorite colorful snacks?*
2. *What are colorful meals you like to share with family and friends?*

Journal

Activity, Not Exercise

You do not need to exercise. I repeat: you do not need to exercise. What? Is this wellness blasphemy? No. "Exercise" is a recent, man-made construction, and the dominant conceptualization is that more is always better. This can make us push our bodies when they need rest. "Exercise" is us telling ourselves we are lazy.

Indeed, we, in a modern world, are not lazy. In fact, we have never worked longer hours at more mentally challenging tasks. The problem is that we are not active. We are hardly lazy, but we are not active. Our minds are getting a workout, but our bodies are exhausted from being slumped over, not doing what they are meant to do—move. Instead, we are "comfortable." We didn't want to walk everywhere, so we invented bikes, and then figured out a way to get to work faster—and with less sweat!—in cars.

It is not natural, though. All that time sitting in cars, desks, and couches is making our bodies feel crummy. Achy and bloated. Physically tired, even though we have not really done anything. Once you start nourishing yourself better, you will likely feel a whole lot more vibrant. Walking to your car at the end of your workday won't feel so far. You are going to be in prime condition to do what you are meant to do: sweat, move, go.

We are animals. We are not plants who can thrive in just one place. Our bodies are made for doing things. The problem is we are doing less and less with our arms and more and more with our thumbs. Sadly, our minds are just telling us over and over that we are lazy and we should go to the gym because our bodies are trying to get us up and out of our chairs.

Still, we don't need to "exercise." We are fancy monkeys, and monkeys don't work out. What then? How do we get physically fit, strong, and shapely, or get the mood boosting exercise compounds, endorphins, coursing through our brains? It's simple: we need to get active. Not so scary, right? Not so hard to commit to.

Commit simply to being active by planning out for yourself when you will fit in time to move. Put it in your planner. Show yourself it is a priority. Perhaps thinking of it as a frequent medical appointment you cannot miss will remind you of how crucial it is to your long-term health. Particularly if you are recovering from addiction or any compulsive behavior, a routine practice of being active can be a crucial way to burn off nervous energy and to feel a grounding, natural high.

Activity can mean literally anything you do that challenges your heart and muscles. Carrying your groceries home in your arms. Gardening. Playing basketball with your kids. Taking a salsa class. Walking your dog. All of these are a lot more palatable than "exercise," right? (Okay, not the first one!)

It's mental. When we tell ourselves we must exercise, we are telling ourselves we need to do some constructed thing that may feel psychologically punitive and generally just sounds hard or boring. Instead, give yourself something to look forward to, consider learning a new hobby (kickboxing, Tai Chi, Zumba), or training for an event, like a race for the cure.

This is so key. It is critical, even, because the primary reason people don't move is either because they dread it or because it sounds like just another responsibility. When we think about being active as something we give ourselves, rather than something taking time away from other priorities, we are far more likely to show up. Signing up for a body pump class probably sounds like a hell of a better time than signing up for a NordicTrack!

That being said, I am not suggesting personal exercise equipment is bad, but that it is not as likely to get used or get you excited.

The people who do use elliptical machines, treadmills, and bikes usually use them at a gym, around other people. They may be enjoying some alone time, listening to their favorite playlist or podcast, but they are doing it in a social setting. Why? Because we are social animals, and we are more likely to push ourselves when together. Seeing others around you doing something healthy will engage you more.

Making movement a social activity helps in two other key ways. First, it makes it simply more fun, and you are more likely to be consistent. Commit to a kick boxing class with a friend, and you will both feel more empowered and be more likely to stick with it. So many of our social experiences center on sitting, so making plans that center on movement can be a healthy new habit in your life. Meet up for a hike, a bike ride, or just a walk in the park. You will feel great and bond in a new way.

Second, if you are predisposed to becoming obsessive and pushing yourself too hard or too long, working out with others can help you recognize normal, healthy limits. You may feel compelled to do three step classes in a row (a sign of exercise bulimia, for example), but chances are that your friends do not. Moving should make you feel vibrant, not weak or dizzy. Pushing yourself when you are exhausted is dangerous. Remember, you are moving to care for yourself, not to burn calories.

Similarly, try to avoid the mindset that being active gives you the freedom to over- indulge. This is a tempting philosophy, but it can be a slippery slope. You should not be working out so you can justify eating unhealthy foods. Instead, think of the movement itself as a source of energy, something you do to give yourself power. Don't undermine that positive effect by counteracting your hard work. Remember the old adage: junk in, junk out.

The bottom line is: you do need to move to thrive. Go ahead and tell yourself your NP said you didn't have to "exercise," if it helps. I love you, whatever amount of weight you can lift. However, if you want to be your most vibrant self, get active. Do whatever is fun, and challenge yourself as much as feels good. If you love marathons, by all means, "Run Forrest! Run!" If you love gardening, then get out there and get your hands dirty. Be an animal, though, and challenge yourself. If you can talk, but only in short sentences, it probably is cardiovascular enough to count as activity. If you can sing, you might not be pushing yourself hard enough to reap the heart-healthy benefits.

Don't minimize the benefits of less strenuous activity, either. Extensive research shows that short episodes of activity added together are just as good, or maybe even better, than long workouts. So, simply build frequent activity into your day. Park farther from the door, take the stairs: every little bit counts. Also, don't discount activities like yoga and Tai Chi, which help you develop strength, flexibility, and balance. All of these are key for preventing injury and feeling centered.

Overall, try to be active every day. Vary what you do to achieve balance, to avoid overstressing your joints and muscles, and simply to avoid boredom. But, whatever you do, move. Move often. Remember, trees are pretty, but you are not a tree. You are a monkey. Monkeys swing.

PRACTICE

Take some time to breathe slowly and deeply for at least a minute, focusing on the sensations of your breath. Then, envision yourself vibrant, strong, and joyful. Use your journal to reflect on the following:

1. *If you were told you could never exert yourself again, what physical activities would you yearn for?*
2. *How can you be more active in a way that feels exciting and fun?*

Journal

Congratulations, you have reviewed all the key principles of Un-Less: Health Begins with Heal; Reasoned, Not Rigid; Soothe; Radiant, Not Clean; Sweetness; Spice; Mindful Dining; Savor; Hunger; Sustain; Satiety; Nourish; Nature; Color; and Activity, Not Exercise.

I hope you have a renewed sense of self-determination and are looking forward to—maybe for the first time in your life—really enjoying yourself. Still, you have lots more to learn (from yourself!), so keep reading and writing. We are just getting started.

PART III

Body Positivity and Self-Love

For many people, self-love is something you have to earn. How often have you thought, *I'll love my stomach when it's flat, my arms when they're sculpted, my hair when it's less frizzy, my mind when it's less scattered?* The problem with this mentality is that you are making your self-love conditional. And, just like the love of your partner, your children, and all those close to you, self-love should be unconditional. Does that mean you have to love the cellulite on your thighs? No. You are free to dislike it. In fact, it may be this discontent that gets you to spinning class when you'd rather watch the game.

On the other hand, body positivity and unconditional self-love mean you do have to *love* your thighs. You have to love them because they are part of you. They enable you to walk, to carry things, to be a person who is able to do the physical tasks that the world presents. In this way, you love your thighs because they are instruments. You may dislike them because they are not your favorite ornaments, but you love them because they enable you to enjoy life. This analogy came to me from a quote by singer Alanis Morissette, who has battled body image issues. Yes, she is the very same woman who did an entire music video naked! Thus, we see that even those who appear to have unbelievable body confidence have had to work at learning to value themselves as more than a series of sexy parts—whatever constitutes sexy this decade!

Once we adopt this idea—that our bodies are instruments and not ornaments—we are able to love ourselves as we are. The changes we seek then become functional, not aesthetic. If you dislike your thighs because they are too weak for you to pick up your child with ease or to be able to take your dog for a nice long walk, then doing squats changes from a move you do to get slim, to the way you enable yourself to thrive. Your goal becomes functional fitness, which is very achievable, rather than image-oriented "health," which may never feel within reach.

I have a family member who is so obese that it is painful for him to walk. Sure, he is not bed-bound like some of the patients I care for, but when he goes to a party, he cannot mingle. He must instead sit somewhere and wait for people to come over to greet him. Far more important than the fact that he doesn't have a six-pack is the fact that his belly is so large that it impedes normal physical tasks, such as tying his own shoes. His body is an instrument that is failing him, an instrument so out of tune (tone) that it no longer allows him to play.

Now, most of you reading this are not in such an extreme state. Your bodies let you do what you want, *to a certain degree*. For example, when I was out of shape, I never had trouble accomplishing my daily tasks. However, when I went on a hike in Yosemite, I found myself much more winded than my friends. My heart was pounding. I was sweating profusely. My legs became so tired that I twisted my knee on a steep decline. I was humiliated because the group had to take frequent breaks for me to rest. I was ashamed that I had let myself get so out of shape. Here I was, in one of the most beautiful places in the world, and I wasn't able to focus on the scenery. I struggled through, step after step. I was sickened by the fact that I had such a hard time on the hike. I had never had an experience before when I was too out of shape to enjoy myself. While I was not obese at that point, I had stopped tuning my instrument, nor was I nourishing myself well. We drank beers as we went down the trail, and my breakfast was a grease-laden breakfast sandwich that leaked oil through the bag. It was not until a couple years after that trip that I decided to dedicate myself to getting healthy. However, it sticks in my mind as one of the crowning experiences that compelled me to treat myself better.

Caring for ourselves is about loving ourselves in the here and now, but it is also about doing what it takes in the long-term to promote wellness. This is a fine balance. We must love our bodies, whatever state they are in, grateful for what they enable us to do. However, we must also nurture them. Indeed, it may be much easier to love your body if you think of it not so much as loving yourself exactly the way you are, but instead as being loving to yourself no matter how out of tune your instrument may be. You do not have to like your belly when it's hanging over your pants, but you must love your stomach for allowing you to grow a baby or carry a suitcase for a long- awaited guest.

Perhaps the simplest way to explain this is to consider your body parts as a system of organs that can be critiqued based on their functionality. They are instruments, not parts to be critiqued based on their appearance, or ornaments. Ornaments are very culturally dictated and change based on the current definition of goodness. For example, it used to be that pale and soft, with little muscle definition, was considered beautiful and classy. Only peasants were out working under the sun, becoming taut, lithe machines. Now, many people would agree, the tanner and more defined, the better—but this is all a social construction.

For example, we have a culturally prescribed notion of a what a good arm is: most likely, the arm is lean and defined. Do any of these things describe the arm's usefulness, though? No. An arm need only be strong enough to carry a normal load, with a wide enough range of motion to reach all the things you need. Thus, when we think of our arms as instruments and not ornaments, we are much easier on ourselves. It is much easier to love your arm when you think of its purpose, not its appearance.

Thinking of yourself as a collection of organs that need to be cared for so they can fulfill their purposes, makes healthy eating and being active a lot more compelling. Even if you have a high metabolism that lets you eat at a bakery every morning without packing on a muffin top, you won't want to start every day with sugar and refined flour when you think of the high-quality energy your instrument needs. Similarly, you know you should not skip meals or exercise despite injury when you think of yourself as an instrument, not an ornament.

Lastly, it may be easier to love your body parts when you use their anatomic names. "Thigh" is very loaded, whereas "hamstring" is not. The first is often sexualized, which instantly means that it is valued based on appearance. The second is wholly valued based on function, not form.

PRACTICE

Take some time to breathe slowly and deeply for at least a minute, focusing on the sensations of your breath. Then, envision yourself vibrant, strong, and joyful. Use your journal to reflect on the following:

1. *What is one part of your body that you may not like but that you can commit to appreciating for what it allows you to do?*
2. *How will you express this body positivity?*

Journal

Health Habits that Unleash Unconditional Wellness

Obesity researchers conducted a landmark study that pooled aggregate data on many thousands of people and found a result that is startling to many people, especially health care providers. They found that five health behaviors were more predictive of wellness than weight.[8] Obese people that were doing well with these behaviors were healthier than normal-weight individuals who were not. In other words, wellness is far more about what you do than what you weigh.

The Five Habits

- Getting seven or more hours of sleep each night
- Eating five or more servings of fruits and vegetables per day
- Exercising at a moderate level of exertion most days of the week for at least thirty minutes
- Drinking light to moderate alcohol (fewer than two drinks per day for men, one for women)
- Not smoking

The great news about the health habits above is that most of them emphasize doing something more, rather than less. This reinforces the Un-Less philosophy, that wellness is about what we can do more of, rather than less of, and that we deserve to give ourselves more. More love. More self-care. More body positivity.

---

8   H. Weisman, "Reducing Weight Stigma." *San Francisco Veterans Healthcare System,* Medical Grand Rounds, 2008.

PRACTICE

Take some time to breathe slowly and deeply for at least a minute, focusing on the sensations of your breath. Then, envision
yourself vibrant, strong, and joyful. Use your journal to reflect on
the following:

1. *Which of these five health habits do you want to do more of?
    Why?*
2. *Which of these five health habits are you already doing well
    with? How can you enhance this strength?*

Journal

Healthy Weight

A key principle of body positivity is that all bodies are respected. Most cultures define beauty, especially female beauty, with being slim. Underneath this is the subtext that women should not "take up too much space" or be too powerful. This is garbage. All people's bodies deserve love and respect. Un-Less is founded on the core principle that we deserve to love ourselves as we are right now, no matter the size and no matter the weight. Indeed, Un-Less also holds that long-term wellness will only occur when we practice self-care rather than self-deprivation or self-criticism. For unconditional wellness, our self-love cannot depend on an outside calculation telling us we are worthy.

That being said, we do know that health is associated with avoiding being under-weight or obese. Both are associated with the risk of disease and poor nutrition. Therefore, it is important to know that, if you do fall into one of these categories, not because you are somehow bad, but because, in order to show yourself love, you may want to change your health habits to improve your wellness. It is also crucial to have an accurate way to know if you are truly under-weight or obese because our culture is so diet-obsessed that many of us walk around feeling bad about ourselves when we are indeed at a perfectly healthy weight.

The best tool for most people to assess if they are at a healthy weight is the waist-to-hip ratio. It is very simple to use and homes in on the fact that the type of adipose (fat) tissue that is risky is abdominal fat, excess weight around your middle. You simply do not want your torso carrying significant weight because excess fat near all your vital organs impairs their function and creates inflammation and risk of disease. Excess abdominal fat, where your body appears more like an apple than a pear, is the concerning type. Conversely, carrying extra weight in your hips and thighs may actually confer some protective benefits. A waist-to-hip ratio of <0.8 is considered low-risk for metabolic diseases such as diabetes, heart disease, and many cancers. It is that simple. Waist-to-hip ratio is a great parameter because people are less likely obsess over insignificant changes that don't reflect real changes in health risk.

On the other hand, if you suspect you may be underweight, you may benefit from finding out your body mass index (BMI), which is weight, in kilograms, divided by height, in centimeters. BMI calculation is known to be less accurate for those with significant muscle mass or who hold their adipose (fat) tissue in their lower body. (As above, that is significantly healthier than having it around your middle.) However, if you have a BMI of less than 22, it indicates that you are below a weight that confers health. You are likely not to be taking in a balanced diet with sufficient nutrients or be maintaining enough muscle mass for strength and vitality. As with everything, moderation is key.

Your Baseline

Wouldn't it be so much more meaningful to know how much better your body is doing with truly robust data? I recommend that if you have a waist-to-hip ratio of >0.8 or a BMI of less than 22, you schedule an overall check-up. I say this not because Un-Less is at all unhealthy, but because I want you to establish a baseline so that, later on, you have more victories to celebrate!

Visit your medical provider and let them know you are beginning a new approach to wellness and want to get baseline tests and evaluate your disease risks. Discuss any issues you know are getting in your way, such as or substance abuse, mental health issues, or family stress. Lay it all on the table. How are you mentally, emotionally, and spiritually? Are you lonely, grieving, worried, anxious, or depressed? Are you feeling hopeless, helpless, fated to be stuck? How often do you feel joy and excitement? Are you smoking, drinking, or using drugs to feel better? What brings you purpose and meaning? What do you want your health for?

In addition to these questions, it is also critical to consider how your body is functioning. Do you feel winded when you walk upstairs? Are you able to walk your dog at a speed to really challenge him? Are you strong enough to put your own bag in the overhead compartment? Do you need a cup of coffee (or three!) every afternoon to get through your day? Does your back ache? Do you suffer from headaches, indigestion, fatigue, or other non-specific symptoms? All in all, how does it feel to live in your body? Do you feel radiant? Being radiant is about far more than any numeric calculation related to your body. Unconditional wellness of mind, body, and spirit cannot be measured.

PRACTICE

Take some time to breathe slowly and deeply for at least a minute, focusing on the sensations of your breath. Then, envision yourself vibrant, strong, and joyful. Use your journal to reflect on the following:

1. *What part of your baseline are you most proud of or grateful for?*
2. *What health concerns do you have, and how do you want to commit to improve your well-being?*

Journal

Journaling the Here and Now

One of the key principles of mindfulness is that we can let go of concerns about the past or future by grounding ourselves in the present and focusing awareness on the here and now.

PRACTICE

Take some time to breathe slowly and deeply for at least a minute, focusing on the sensations of your breath. Then, envision yourself vibrant, strong, and joyful. Use your journal to reflect on at least three of the following:

1. *Your Present*
   a. What is going on right now in your life that is making it hard to be healthy?
   b. What can you do to minimize, eliminate, or modify these challenges?
   c. What are you doing right now that will help you get healthier?
   d. How can you emphasize or increase this?
   e. Who can you reach out to for support? Emotional? Mental? Financial? Physical? Practical?
   f. Why is today a great day to start taking better care of yourself?
   g. What motivates you to take better care of your body?
   h. What benefits are you discovering by improving your relationship with food?
   i. What spiritual and emotional factors help boost your dedication to nourishing yourself?
   j. Who is your wellness role model? Why?

k. What benefits are you feeling by increasing your self-care?

l. What healthy foods do you love?

m. What physical activities do you enjoy? How can you do more of them?

n. What does your body allow you to do that you are grateful for?

o. What do you need to apologize to your body for?

Journal

Me-Time

The classic book *Men Are from Mars, Women Are from Venus* asserts that women are most loving to others when they feel good about themselves.[9] When feeling down on themselves, they are hard on others as well. I doubt this is a true reflection of women only. It is true for me, as well as everyone else I know, male or female. Similarly, it is said that one way to glean if someone is depressed is whether they make you feel depressed when you are around them. Simply put, negative feelings are contagious. Feeling consistently bad about yourself and the world around you makes others feel unable to help, critical, and pessimistic.

So, what does this imply? That if you're depressed you're a terrible friend? Or, that you should drop all of your friends who are blue in order to live happily? No. If you are depressed, you will fare much better with a strong support network. Similarly, if you can focus on the needs of others, when necessary, you can be a great, extra-sympathetic, friend. Comforting others and cheering them up, when possible, may in fact make you feel better in turn. You feel useful, responsible, and capable, all empowering feelings. However, it can also be quite draining to cheer up those around you, whether it be through "being strong," hearing them out when they need to vent, or helping them think positively. It's virtually impossible to be the life raft all the time: with enough weight piled upon you, you will deflate.

How, then, can we stay afloat, all while being the compassionate reliable people we want to be? How can we ensure that, while caring for parents, children, spouses, and friends, we do not undermine our own wellness? It's simple: we must make time to refresh

---

9   J. Gray, *Men Are from Mars, Women Are from Venus*. (New York, New York: HarperCollins, 1992)

ourselves. One friend calls this being "healthfish" to remind herself that it is not selfish, but healthy.

Typically, you hear the phrase "me-time" in one of three contexts. First, it's used to describe the time you need for self-care. This may take the form of a work-out, a chance to look for a more fulfilling job, or the opportunity to do whatever you need to do to assure yourself long-term success. I call this form of me-time the "long look." If neglected, you risk living too much for the moment, always prioritizing the here and now, and missing out on how to care for the future.

The second kind of me-time might be best described as pampering. Here you give yourself a manicure, take a long bath, or enjoy a long afternoon on the golf course, without regard for the chores waiting at home. This is an indulgence that allows you to be present in your senses and bask in whatever feels good. Indeed, we actually need feel-good sensory experiences, and, when we deny them, they will assert themselves. If this type of me-time is neglected, you risk giving into momentary pleasures which are not so healthy: overeating, drinking, smoking, risky sex. Overall, if we don't allow ourselves to bask in whatever healthy sensory experiences we crave—skydiving anyone?—we risk falling prey to a much less healthy rush.

A third kind of me-time is the type that is unstructured, unscheduled, unscripted. This is time to daydream. It may take the form of a calm cup of coffee in the morning, when the house is quiet, before responsibilities set in. It may be a leisurely walk with the dog, aimless, following the sights and sounds you see. Perhaps it's taking a bath until your toes get pruney, without multi-tasking. No reading a book, no texting, no dyeing your hair. In fact, this is the anti-multi-tasking. It means giving yourself time in which you seek to accomplish nothing. You seek nothing. You just bask and let your mind go. When was the last time you just lay in the grass and watched the clouds? Basked in the sun and just thought about the light shining on you?

Even recreational activities can engage our minds in a way that takes us away from our own thoughts. When was the last time you just drove without listening to the radio, or sat on the couch without watching TV? While it may be wonderful to hear the news around the world or watch a romantic comedy, it does take away from the time that your mind has a chance to explore your own hopes, wishes, dreams, and inspirations. Each time you tune into media, you are choosing to think other people's thoughts!

Perhaps this is why I have come up with some of my most creative ideas while doing things that are not mentally stimulating in any way—using the elliptical, grooming horses, cleaning the bathroom. It is in these times that your mind is free to wander—that is, if you let it. If you're making phone calls or doing anything else that takes your mind away, you have re-engaged with the world. In this last form of me-time, you are disengaging. You are pulling the plug on all electronics, getting off the grid. Try to quiet the voice in your mind that tells you to focus on the task at hand. Instead, just reflect on your own life. Maybe this is why many people have an increasing need for therapy: they do not take the time to reflect on their lives otherwise. Their minds are always focused outwardly rather than inwardly.

You may ask which form of me-time is the most important. The long-term self-care, pampering, or time to daydream? The answer is all three. All forms of me-time are necessary to get the most out of life. Remember, being loving towards yourself allows you to be loving to others. Allowing yourself me-time assures that you can give off positive energy, which usually brings positive energy back to you!

If it feels overwhelming to squeeze in all three forms, reflect on which sounds the most alluring to you, and put it into your schedule. It need not be a long period. Taking a few minutes for a walk before you rush home from work takes maybe twenty minutes, but putting on a playlist that pumps you up before getting in the shower takes only one. The point is not to make you feel even more overscheduled, but to fit in time for you in your life. Indeed, take this as license to start cancelling whatever is not critically necessary and/or doesn't bring you joy. When we care for ourselves, we are more loving to others because we need not be resentful. We don't *need* those around us because we have already met our own basic needs. We are therefore empowered to *choose* what we want.

Your ultimate goal is likely to be a good mother, father, daughter, brother, friend. Once you internalize that it is good, even necessary, to make time for your own needs, the sooner you can achieve this goal. You will find yourself less snippy, more accepting. You will allow others to take the time to care for themselves, as well, and they will be ever grateful. It seems illogical, but caring for yourself is actually a gift you give to others. This is often expressed as caring for yourself physically, so you can live a long, healthy life, but it can also be a short-term gift. By devoting the time you need to prepare for your future, live for the moment, and let your mind be open, you show others that they, too, deserve self-care.

You may find it challenging to put your own needs first because you were taught that your child's, partner's, or parent's needs are more important. What would happen if your daughter did not grow up with this perspective? Might she be more able to insist on safe sex? Less willing to accept abuse from a partner? Overall, be more capable of standing up for herself?

PRACTICE

Take some time to breathe slowly and deeply for at least a minute, focusing on the sensations of your breath. Then, envision yourself vibrant, strong, and joyful. Use your journal to reflect on the following:

1. *How would you like to spend your next "long look" session? Next pampering period? Next day dreaming time?*

Journal

PART IV

What is Healthy Eating?

Healthy eating depends only partially on eating healthy food. In addition to making sure you give your body quality energy, the act of eating, or, again, dining, should be one that is holistically healthy—that cares for your mind and spirit. Thus, Un-Less is about a lot more than biochemistry. It is about being mindful of the fact that eating is perhaps the only act that you do multiple times a day, every day, that has social, psychological, political, and environmental effects. If you are like me, the more mindful you are about how you eat, the more mindful you will become about all the choices you make.

Un-Less offers a contemplative way of being, that knows that the heart of health is being close to and respectful of nature. Science should guide consideration, but, remember, there is no scientific formula to follow. Instead, you must follow your intuition and let go of the seductive illusion of perfectionism. This approach allows you to be flexible, easy going, and spontaneous, which opens you up to being able to enjoy all that the world offers.

Un-Less asserts that you can be trusted to figure out a way of eating that keeps you healthy, and that you don't need rules! The approach stands firm against the notion that there is a singular prescription for health. Becoming healthy is a journey and means different things for different people because we each have different goals.

Feeling frustrated? Feeling like I tricked you into reading a book that would teach you about healthy eating and then asserted that there's no clear-cut way? Fear not. The difference between this approach and any other you've tried before is that I offer you principles, and you choose which ones to focus on. You can be a vegetarian. You can be a burger fanatic. (Grass-fed beef can have as many inflammation-fighting omega threes as fish!) You can swear by milk. You can drink only almond milk. These things don't really matter in the big picture. Un-Less is bigger than these details. The approach is, first and foremost, about improving your relationship with food and body image, so that you can mindfully choose which ways of eating suit your unique mind and spirit. You can have great success, through reason, not rigidity.

PRACTICE

Take some time to breathe slowly and deeply for at least a minute, focusing on the sensations of your breath. Then, envision yourself vibrant, strong, and joyful. Use your journal to reflect on the following:

1. *How would you describe a healthy eating behavior?*
2. *What eating habits have you had in the past that did not reflect unconditional self-love? How can you change these habits?*

Journal

Tips for Being Healthy on the Go

Being healthy can be easier at home, where you have more influence over food, company, ambience, and timing. But you do not belong at home, at least not all the time.

Learning to nourish yourself on the go is an art. It requires planning, such as bringing healthy snacks, but it also requires practicing all the mindfulness that keeps your energy positive, calm, and creative. Keep it simple for yourself by making the easy choice the healthy one. For example, in terms of eating, surround yourself with a variety of nutritious foods, not just one snack. It will stop you from feeling deprived, and it is a good way to remind yourself that food is not an enemy. Stock your office and car with a few items, from different food groups, that will provide balance and novelty, such as almonds, dried fruit, turkey jerky, and hard-boiled eggs. These foods are all easy to find at gas stations and corner stores!

In terms of movement, make it simple to be active. Join the gym that is closest to your office or home, so you don't have to go out of your way to get strong. Set up dates, such as hiking and dance classes, with friends that are active, so you never have to decide between being social and being fit. Set up meetings with colleagues where you walk, at least to the coffee shop down the street. Being away from your desks will invigorate you and may make you more collaborative and innovative. Buy three yoga mats so you can always unwind at a moment's notice. Keep one in your car, one at home, and one in your office. Get small weights so that, even when you couldn't make it to a workout, you can do some curls after dinner while chatting with family. Don't have space in your home to do squats? Go on your porch or your roof. Being active outdoors may boost your energy and will better regulate your circadian rhythm to improve sleep and help your body create vitamin D from the sun. Fifteen minutes per day without sunscreen is essential for the development of this vital nutrient, which is necessary for bone health, mood, blood sugar regulation, and may decrease the risk of some cancers.

When you travel, look for active ways to adventure, to help your digestion of local treats, and to keep yourself positive when there are snags along the way. Choose the hotel with the pool where you could actually swim laps or go to the gym when you are up at 4:00 am from jet lag.

Overall, make it easy for yourself to make a healthy choice. Remember, being healthy is a gift you give yourself and your loved ones. Carry your journal, so you can always be reflective. When in doubt, call a friend who reminds you of why you want to make positive changes for yourself.

PRACTICE

Take some time to breathe slowly and deeply for at least a minute, focusing on the sensations of your breath. Then, envision yourself vibrant, strong, and joyful. Use your journal to reflect on the following:

1. *What are ways for you to practice mindful dining at your workplace?*
2. *What about when visiting with family?*

Journal

The Trouble with Tipsy

Drinking alcohol can have significant health benefits, be it in the form of wine, beer, or even hard liquor. Metabolizing alcohol has been shown to help balance blood sugar levels, and some alcohol contains certain antioxidants which help with heart health and prevent cancer and promote longevity. So, no need to swear off booze with Un-Less.

However, these benefits are only shown to exist for light to moderate drinkers, and moderate is defined as an average of two drinks per day for men and one for women. This does not mean seven drinks on Saturday night, ladies! A serving of wine is 4 ounces, a serving of beer is 12 ounces, and a serving of liquor is one ounce. So, chances are, from a medical standpoint, you are a heavier drinker than you think. If you are able to be a light to moderate drinker, go right ahead and continue your ways. I toast to you.

For others, changing your relationship with alcohol may be a key way to nourish yourself. If you have ever tried cutting back but had difficulty, and especially if you have had ongoing personal, professional, or legal problems as a result of your drinking, please consult a healthcare professional or support group. Many people are able to make it past alcohol abuse and dependence and lead rich and exciting lives. The same goes for drugs.

I personally do not have difficulty with abusing substances. When I do drink, I thankfully have that off-switch that signals to me "enough is enough," and I generally listen. That being said, when I drink, my natural personality becomes more extreme. I am already a social butterfly, but I then become distractible and less considerate of others. Sometimes, after a party, I feel I just bounced around and did not really savor any of my conversations. Also, I am much more likely to make poor eating choices and not tune into my body about when it is hungry or full, munching mindlessly on junk food or grabbing candy at the corner store. These are not problems once in a while, but they can become unhealthy patterns.

PRACTICE

Take some time to breathe slowly and deeply for at least a minute, focusing on the sensations of your breath. Then, envision yourself vibrant, strong, and joyful. Use your journal to reflect on the following:

1. *How does alcohol affect your eating choices?*
2. *How can you have a healthier relationship to alcohol or drugs?*

Journal

Chronic Pain

There are few things worse than chronic pain. When you are in pain, it becomes very alluring to eat for comfort. You may even be scared to move, for fear of worsening the pain. As such, many of my patients with chronic pain struggle with obesity. Unfortunately, the obesity exacerbates the pain, creating a vicious cycle. How can it be broken?

I myself struggle with chronic neck and upper back pain, a result of an old injury and car accident, exacerbated by being busty. At its worst, it was a 9/10, leading me to stand rather than sit to get through class and requiring opiate pain medications and frequent trips to an osteopath specializing in spinal manipulation. Now, it is managed by eating an anti-inflammatory diet, getting chiropractic adjustments and acupuncture when needed, staying active so I am strong and flexible, and taking an over-the-counter anti-inflammatory (naproxen) once in a while. What does this show? Basically, that I have tried most non-pharmacologic and pharmacologic (medication-based) treatments. I am even considering surgical intervention, since a breast reduction would likely improve the problem, as well. This is what I recommend to you, too—NP's orders: try all the modalities recommended to you. They work best together. Consult both conventional and integrative providers, who can combine evidence-based complementary and alternative treatments.

That is what I have always told my husband, too. He has severe Degenerative Disc Disease and has already had three major surgeries at a young age. Although these were required for reduction of his symptoms, his long-term management includes anti- inflammatory medications and botanicals, stretching, and maintaining strength and weight, massage, chiropractic therapy, and acupuncture. In other words, he has taken control of the pain and done what is needed to feel good.

I share these stories because I want you to see that I, as a human being, as a wife, and as a provider, understand the complexity of chronic pain. For many sufferers whose conditions are progressive, the pain will be never ending. It can always be better managed, though, and looking broadly at all the things you can do is empowering. If your pain has a neurologic (nerve) component, certain anti-depressants or even anti-epileptic drugs may be useful, due to their stabilizing effect on pain-related neuro-transmitters. The short answer is: there is help.

Lastly, I cannot stress enough the value of healthy eating when it comes to chronic pain. Highly processed foods have been shown to have inflammatory effects, and inflammation is the root of most pain. Eating in a way that minimizes inflammation is key, and right now there is booming research on reducing inflammation naturally with botanicals. You would be wise to seek out more information beyond the scope of this book.

Overall, however, remember that a natural diet rich in antioxidants, plants, protein and healthy fats is a great jumping off point, and reaching and maintaining a healthy weight reduces inflammation throughout your body. It can even prevent the development of some cancers and absolutely prevents diabetes and heart disease.

Lastly, care for your mental and emotional health. Pain takes an enormous toll on your mood and your relationships. Therapy can be very useful in this realm. Coping better emotionally may help you use your pain treatments more effectively and feel more motivation to make useful changes to your diet and otherwise. Therapy, meditation, and yoga may help you reframe your relationship with the discomfort and make you feel more empowered.

In sum, consider the problem holistically. Nourish yourself, be proactive, creative, and open minded, and you can take control of your pain. Consider working with a whole team of professionals to get your pain managed better. There is always more that can be done.

PRACTICE

Take some time to breathe slowly and deeply for at least a minute, focusing on the sensations of your breath. Then, envision yourself vibrant, strong, and joyful. Use your journal to reflect on the following:

1. *How does pain or other discomfort affect your health choices?*
2. *What have you done in the past that helps, and how can you enhance this?*

Journal

Beauty Sleep

Now that we have discussed all the things you must do to nourish yourself, let's discuss what you should not do. Do not move for seven to ten hours per day. What? For most people this is the ideal amount of sleep. Sleep is crucial for memory, concentration, energy, and—simply—beauty. Do you want to be a radiant super-hero? Go to bed.

In our busy lives, sleep can seem like the lowest priority. It is easy to try to burn the candle at both ends and eke out another hour of the day by reducing sleep. However, you will always lose in the end. Low mental performance and emotional instability make any additional work hours less productive and efficient. And getting less than seven hours per night of sleep chronically is associated with dysregulation of hormones and related weight gain. Sleep is nature's way of taking the time it needs to heal itself. Do not mess with it.

If you struggle with insomnia, as I have, try everything you can before turning to prescription sleep aides. They are high in abuse potential and can have severe side effects. Even seemingly harmless over-the-counter compounds can be very dangerous for seniors. Benadryl, or diphenhydramine, which many people take for sleep, can create wakefulness and agitation and lead to falls. For some people, natural sleep remedies can be very useful. Valerian and mela-tonin are both natural compounds with very little risk that can be effective and safe for most everyone. Talk to your medical provider or pharmacist.

Before these sleep aides, there are many other things to try. First, what we call Sleep Hygiene. These are all the non-pharmaco-logic practices that help your body relax and go to sleep naturally. Avoid stimulating activities at night, especially in the last hour. The worst culprits are screens, such as TVs, computers, and smart phones, which emit a wavelength called "blue light" which is very stimulating to the brain. Also, avoid eating shortly before bed, since this is activating. Do quiet, relaxing things, like taking a bath, folding laundry, reading a book, meditating, or praying. *Yoga Nidra* is a meditative yoga that is very helpful for insomnia and many downloads are available free, online. If it calms you, masturbate, or make love. If you have trouble quieting your mind, especially regarding your responsibilities, make a list of the things you need to get done the next day to let your mind know you will come back to them. If you still remain lying in bed awake longer than about thirty minutes (what we call normal sleep "latency"), then read or get out of bed and do something boring, like folding laundry. Just lying there getting frustrated that you cannot sleep makes it worse. Do not turn on the TV and start a Netflix binge.

PRACTICE

Take some time to breathe slowly and deeply for at least a minute, focusing on the sensations of your breath. Then, envision yourself vibrant, strong, and joyful. Use your journal to reflect on the following:

1. *What can you do to improve your sleep hygiene habits?*
2. *What is limiting the healing power of sleep in your life?*

Journal

Vibrant Spirit

For many people, spirituality is a robust, core part of life. For others, just the word spirituality can be off-putting and anxiety-producing. Un-Less considers spiritual practices any beliefs or behaviors that give you a sense of wonder, purpose, strength, connectedness, and hope. You may have a spiritual connection to a synagogue, mosque, or church, or to nature, meditation, or poetry. Whatever you do, though, make your spiritual health a priority. Engage in rituals or habits that remind you that we have a deep consciousness that allows us to show ourselves and the world a deep empathy. I personally believe that when we act with empathy, with compassion, that is a holy act. When we uplift ourselves and each other, we are therefore acting with holiness. However you define spirituality, I hope it brings you purpose and meaning and leads you to compassion.

In sum, I am a modern yogi from California. I believe there is wisdom in every religion but that religion is often also used throughout the world to justify discrimination and uphold the status quo. So, I lean towards just following the Golden Rule: do unto others as you would do unto yourself. However, I often see people treat others better than they treat themselves. So, instead, I say, "Namaste," which is often defined as, "I see and honor the light within you." No matter your beliefs, I hope you can say *amen* to that. In case you don't know, amen means "I agree." I think we can all agree that we should treat our bodies, if not like temples, at least deserving of tender loving care.

PRACTICE

Take some time to breathe slowly and deeply for at least a minute, focusing on the sensations of your breath. Then, envision yourself vibrant, strong, and joyful. Use your journal to reflect on the following:

1. *What kinds of activities give you meaning and purpose?*
2. *How can you use these activities to promote wellness and unconditional self-love?*

Journal

Building Support

Un-Less is safe for everyone, forever. It is pleasurable. It is the anti-diet, and unlike a diet, you are not going to feel jealous of others or get isolated. You can share a tasty meal, a walk, a day at the park. You may feel more liberated and joyful than ever before, and you will likely attract people to you, both physically and emotionally.

That being said, embracing Un-Less means taking a very close and somewhat painful look at your life. When I discuss the approach with people, I am reminded time and again how difficult body issues can be. Even those who have never had eating disorders and have never been obese light up and then tear up. They thank me, grateful for a new, kinder way to live that they can actually relax and enjoy. It will be key to surround yourself with supportive, kind people as you do some soul searching. It will also help if you schedule in some light silliness, so you can let go of that "work" mentality that you might have used before to try to improve your health.

Building a community of friends and family to support you with Un-Less will not be hard. People may not recognize any changes right away, but they will be asking, "What did you do? You look fabulous! Did you go on vacation?!" Share with them the principles of the approach. Get them a copy of the book, and call a week later to ask them how it's going. Talk about what you have been most inspired by. Go over how you are applying each of the principles. Putting it in your own words will help you better understand and integrate the concepts and make the approach feel even more natural. Lastly, you never know: you may be helping someone with a hidden disease or disorder start the path towards healing. Or, you may find out they have struggled in ways you never knew, and you can learn from each other's successes.

Lastly, Un-Less will give you a new awareness of your own feelings and needs. You may recognize that you need to do some significant work to improve relationships with those around you. Taking ownership of past mistakes and poor behavior can be a great first step to making amends. Some relationships may be better terminated than worked on, depending on how challenging they have become or how willing the other person is to making change. Either way, remember that your relationship with yourself is of primary importance. If you don't honor your own needs, you will not be able to manifest your full vibrant potential.

PRACTICE

Take some time to breathe slowly and deeply for at least a minute, focusing on the sensations of your breath. Then, envision yourself vibrant, strong, and joyful. Use your journal to reflect on the following:

1. *What relationships in your life promote wellness?*
2. *What can you do to strengthen these bonds and enhance this benefit?*

Journal

PART V

Journaling on Mindful Dining and Activity

Congratulations, you have spent time immersing yourself in the heart of Un-Less. You have learned the philosophical principles and learned how to reflect on the past to change your future. You have considered the impact of body positivity, making time for yourself, and how weight actually does, and does not, affect health. You have also delved into what healthy eating behaviors are. Armed with all this knowledge, you can now begin keeping track of your eating behaviors and movement.

This part of the approach comes at the end to emphasize that the focus is not on critiquing yourself, but instead on learning about yourself, and the habits and foods will nourish you. If we did not start with pledging to love ourselves no matter what, this approach would be just another thing you would try to be perfect at. Now you know, there is no formula for success. There is instead a way to discover within yourself what you need to feel peaceful and strong, inside and out. Try not to become obsessed with every bite you put in your mouth. The goal is simply to become more mindful about the physical, mental, emotional, and spiritual components of your eating.

Start with using the hunger scale, from zero to three. Remember: zero is not at all hungry, one is somewhat hungry, two is moderately hungry, and three is ravenous.

Then, consider the social, temporal, physical, and emotional components of your eating habits. Utilize the old journalist's trope: who, what, when, where, and why/how. Who are you with? What are you doing? When is it? Where are you? How do you feel physically and emotionally?

First, the who. Consider the role of others. Are you alone, with your spouse or partner, with a new love, a date, a friend, an acquaintance? Who makes you feel accepted? Who makes you excited? Who might make you feel like you have to diet? Who makes you feel like you should indulge, perhaps so they feel the license to do so as well? Do certain people make comments about your eating that make you uncomfortable? Why? How can you steer the conversation to feel safe or more fulfilling?

Second, the what. Note what you are doing. Are you simply dining, the goal? Or, are you scrolling through Facebook or watching TV, disconnecting from your own experience? Are you working, hammering away at a deadline? What you are doing while you eat affects pace, how much you can savor your food, and whether you will stay tuned into your hunger cues. Whenever possible, stop and dine, whether it is on a park bench or even just in your car.

Third, the when. Note when you eat. This will tune you into your patterns temporally. Do you tend to skip breakfast, have only coffee or juice, and then snack throughout the morning? Or, do you have a big breakfast because you wake up famished since you try not to eat at all at night? Do you eat lunch right at noon or another "appropriate" hour because you feel it's time, even if you're not actually hungry? Do you wait until others are home to eat dinner, but end up stuffing yourself because you've been hungry for hours? Do you not let yourself eat something until after you work out? Do you feel like you have to go work out the moment you eat something "bad"?

Fourth, the where. Where you are eating? In the break room at work? In the car? Standing up at the kitchen counter? At the drive-thru? At your desk? In your dining room? In restaurants? In bars? In class? In bed? On the couch? Which of these places make you feel safe? Which are mentally or emotionally stressful? Where are you focused on your food? Where are you distracted from your meal?

Fifth, the why/how. Write how you feel physically. Feeling lightheaded from waiting too long to eat? Feeling vibrant and strong?

Do you have discomfort? Where and why? How might this be related to pain, exercise, stress, or other triggers?

Paying attention to how you feel physically also identifies any symptoms you might be having of food sensitivities. Ironically, people often crave the foods their bodies do not tolerate or digest well. Eat cheese at every opportunity, but suffering from gas, bloating, and either diarrhea or constipation? Perhaps you are sensitive to dairy products. Being mindful can be downright practical!

In addition, write how you feel emotionally. Pay special attention to the circumstances when you eat. Is something triggering you? Are you nervous? Bored? Missing an ex? Do you have a project that feels overwhelming? Generally, you should eat when you feel calm and collected. Do whatever you need to do to help yourself relax before you start eating, so that you know you are not eating to calm or distract yourself, but to nourish yourself.

All of the sections above help you reflect on your eating behaviors. This is beneficial for most everyone. You can also add what you ate, but only if you think it could be helpful for you and not lead to obsessive thinking. Skip this part if you have a tendency to categorize certain foods as bad and off-limits, which can lead to a diet mindset. Noting what you did eat can help, though, if you find your energy levels to be very unstable or if you have difficulty choosing nourishing foods. You may find reflecting on the food itself can help you see patterns in how different choices affect your physical, mental, and emotional state. If you choose to, you could also count general servings of food types. For example, you could note you had three servings of fruit in your fruit salad. When you note patterns over time, this can help you consider whether you are giving your body all of the types of foods it needs. I strongly recommend against counting calories, which creates an attitude that less is more. This is Un-Less. You are learning to obsess less and love yourself more. Calorie counting does not promote body positivity.

In addition to reflecting on your eating, write down what activity you get. Give yourself credit for everything: gardening for an hour, vigorously cleaning for ten minutes, making love for half an hour. None of these would classically count as exercise, but that is why exercise is a limiting concept. They can all be good ways to challenge your body, build muscle, and get oxygen and happy chemicals, such as serotonin, flowing. While an actual work-out is the best way to get your body strong and fit, writing down all your activity can be encouraging, and may even prove to you that you like being active and are ready to challenge yourself more!

After all this data, conclude your writing with anything else that helps you cultivate gratitude, relax, grow, and feel inspired.

In summary, use your journal to reflect on your eating behaviors for the next few weeks, or however long you continue to learn new things from yourself. Keep track of the following:

1. Start with using the hunger scale, from zero to three.
2. Consider the social, temporal, physical, and emotional components of your eating habits—Who, What, When, Where, Why/How?
   a. Who are you with?
   b. What are you doing?
   c. What time is it?
   d. Where are you?
   e. How do you feel physically? How do you feel emotionally?
3. What are you eating? (Include this only if it does not lead to obsessive thinking.)
4. What movement and activity have you done?

5. What do you feel grateful for?

PRACTICE

Take some time to breathe slowly and deeply for at least a minute, focusing on the sensations of your breath. Then, envision yourself vibrant, strong, and joyful. Use your journal to reflect on the following:

1. *What are you enjoying most about the journaling process?*
2. *What have you been surprised by when you put your thoughts onto paper?*

Journal

Creating Long Term Change

We all know change does not happen overnight, and yet who is not lured by the power of a get-rich-quick scheme? Similarly, we all hope change will be linear, that once we commit to a new way of being, we'll never slip up and make the same mistakes again. Simply put, if change were that easy, you would have done it by now.

Prochaska's widely acclaimed Trans-Theoretical Model of Change is different.[10] It is a model which shows that change is not linear but actually a spiraling cycle and that your progression depends on learning from your normal, predictable mistakes.

Here is an example. Let's imagine a smoker, Alice. Like all smokers, she knows it is bad for her, but yet she is not at all engaging with the thought of quitting. She is in the Pre- Contemplative Phase, just living her life, not concerned about her habit, maybe even loving it.

The next phase is the Contemplative Phase. Here, she starts to think about how she should quit, or at least cut back. She considers why (preventing disease, saving money, smelling better, avoiding wrinkles), but makes no plan, and takes no action.

She may linger in the Contemplative Phase for months or years, or she may return to the Pre-Contemplative Phase, not reflecting on why change is beneficial, prioritizing other things. On the other hand, she also could enter the Planning Phase, strategizing about how to quit. Reading up on tips and tricks, asking friends, buying Nicorette. She may delay the change, saying, "I will quit after I finish this assignment at work," but really the change has already begun, and she has taken action to begin a new way.

10   J. Prochaska and W. Velicer, "The transtheoretical model of health behavior change," *American Journal of Health Promotion* 12, no. 1 (1997): 38-48.

Then again, she could get distracted, and return to the Contemplative Phase, or even the Pre-Contemplative phase. In this way, it is cyclical, like a spring winding forward that can coil off and wind back at any time. Still, she is always farther ahead than if she had never started. If her planning is successful, she enters the Action Phase, her first days without smoking. They may feel unnatural, requiring tremendous focus to sustain. This is the phase that requires the most effort and where most people start to get in their own way. They think about all the reasons they miss it and why change really isn't that important, at least not right now. Alice might see people smoking and laughing, jealous over their easy bond, and her long-term reasons for quitting may feel a lot less seductive.

Still, if she can stick with her plan, she will move forward to the Maintenance Phase, where it is no longer so hard to turn down a cigarette, where she discovers other relaxing habits work better, or, at least, are guilt-free, and she starts to enjoy the benefits and focuses on these. Still, maintenance can be the trickiest phase. After the initial novelty has worn off, the memory of how hard it was to quit fades away. It may become easier to think, "Just one cigarette. I can have one. That is no big deal."

And then she does: she grabs a smoke and lights up. But here is where Prochaska's model is different. When she reverts, she is not a failure. Instead, she is only a "failure" if she smokes and never again tries to quit. If, however, she throws out the pack and starts strategizing again about what to do differently, then she is actually a poster child for real-life change.

The key is using mistakes as learning opportunities in which you see what worked for you, what didn't, and why. You examine your own triggers, and you make plans that incorporate new techniques to strengthen your weaknesses. Does this sound like journaling with

Un-Less? It is. Basically, I am assuming that in your life, you have been through these cycles before with your own wellness. Un-Less can help you through the inevitable pitfalls and help you cycle faster towards well-being.

So, if Alice starts contemplating and planning again, she will likely be in these phases for a much shorter time. She will go right back into action, and then her attempts at maintenance will be more robust. She will know better what she needs to succeed. She will not underestimate how hard it will be. And she will fight for it.

If she is more successful this time, she will enter another phase I coin the Integration Phase (Prochaska ends with Maintenance), where quitting starts to feel like the "new normal." She no longer has to work at it, and new habits replace the function of smoking. Coffee brings her together with friends. Knitting gives her something to do with her nervous energy. Writing songs relaxes her.

So, Un-Less is not built on a model of change that is dichotomous. There is no success or failure because there are no rules to break or choices that are bad or good. Instead, this approach depends on self-analysis because every one of us has different patterns we should change to thrive. We have different skills, passions, struggles, and strengths. Your version of Un-Less is different than mine. Different from Alice's. And yet, they are all the same.

PRACTICE

Take some time to breathe slowly and deeply for at least a minute, focusing on the sensations of your breath. Then, envision yourself vibrant, strong, and joyful. Use your journal to reflect on the following:

1. *What kinds of change have you been contemplating?*
2. *What could help you begin taking action?*
3. *What kinds of change have you undertaken that you want to work on maintaining?*

Journal

Journaling to Strategize for the Future

PRACTICE

Take some time to breathe slowly and deeply for at least a minute, focusing on the sensations of your breath. Then, envision yourself vibrant, strong, and joyful.

Use your journal to reflect on the following:

Your Future

a. Make a collage of photos or images that remind you about nourishing yourself.

b. Make a timeline of goals for yourself for the next day, week, month, and year.

c. Write a letter to children that you love. Share with them what you want them to know about caring for themselves.

d. Write a letter to your future self. Remind yourself of the values you believe in that anchor your wellness.

e. Write your own eulogy. Make it a light-hearted tribute to your wellness legacy and all the things you want to accomplish in the years to come.

Journal

Conclusion

As I write this, I am literally moved to tears reflecting on all the steps it has taken me to get to this point: from harming and then healing my own body and spirit, to learning what it takes to motivate myself, my family, friends, and patients. Our relationship with our bodies is so complex, and, just like every relationship, it will have its ups and downs, periods of crazy love, and crazy fury. What I hope for you, and for everyone, is that it is a healthy relationship: one that may be imperfect but whole; one that drives you to improve but accepts your faults; one that says, "I'm sorry" more often than "I'm right."

Moving past the point of rules and rigidity is critical for real nourishment. Moving past over-indulgence and inertia is critical for real radiance. Whether you have been neglecting yourself by not letting yourself embrace all life has to offer or by trying to soothe your aching heart by filling your belly, you have been holding yourself back. Today is the day to start carrying yourself forward. And in the words of E.E. Cummings, "I carry your heart. I carry it in my heart."[11]

You have reached the end of Un-Less, but your path to body positivity, wellness, and unconditional self-love are just beginning. You have gotten to know your default thoughts and habits, and, by using mindfulness, you have charted a new path to well-being that is unique to you. I have no doubt that this has been a hard journey. It can be frightening to let go of the illusions of security that the diet mindset offers. The diet mindset tells you what is good, bad, clean, dirty, safe, and dangerous. But, as we know, the diet mindset is, at best, unsustainable and, at worst, destructive. No one should live to be clean, just as no one should live to be safe. Life is so much more than eating for nutrition or exercising for cardiovascular benefit.

11   E.E. Cummings. *Complete Poems: 1904-1962*.

We are not simple organisms who just need the correct formula for growth. Instead, we are complex beings with a sophisticated nervous system capable of experiencing pleasure. We radiate heat, and, therefore, we are literally little beacons of light in the world. Un-Less is here to help you find your own wellness wavelength. Shine on.

PRACTICE

Take some time to breathe slowly and deeply for at least a minute, focusing on the sensations of your breath. Then, envision yourself vibrant, strong, and joyful. Use your journal to reflect on the following:

1. *How does Un-Less help you feel more free?*
2. *How does it help you feel more secure?*

Journal

PART VI

Appendix 1: Fifty Cheap, Healthy Ways to Self-Soothe

1. Cuddle with animals.
2. Play with children.
3. Give yourself a "cooking lesson" from a cookbook.
4. Ask an older family member to teach you a favorite recipe.
5. FaceTime a friend you have lost touch with.
6. Make an apology.
7. Accept an apology.
8. Do yoga.
9. Write a thank you note.
10. Write a poem.
11. Write a letter.
12. Send post cards to 10 friends far away.
13. Visit a family member you need to make time for.
14. Volunteer.
15. Give yourself a spa day. Take a bath. Do a manicure and pedicure. Use products, like masks, you never make time for.
16. Play with make up or change your facial hair.
17. Try a new hair style.
18. Plan your next Halloween costume.
19. Go to a thrift store.
20. Donate clothes and other things to de-clutter your home. Let go of things that no longer bring you joy.
21. Plan a date or party.
22. Spend the gift cards you have.
23. Organize your closet.
24. Make your bed and then take a nap.
25. Light a candle and visualize your dream vacation.

26. Put on a favorite album and dance.

27. Play video games.

28. Go for a hike.

29. Stroll through your neighborhood and window shop.

30. Strike up a conversation with a friendly stranger.

31. Look at old photos.

32. Read old letters.

33. Read a book.

34. Sing in the shower.

35. Meditate or pray.

36. Browse in the bookstore.

37. Tend to your plants.

38. Have a glass of wine or another drink, but really savor it.

39. Invite a neighbor over for tea.

40. Go for a walk.

41. Look up free events in your town.

42. Plan your next vacation.

43. Just lie on the ground and look at the sky.

44. Make a list of things you're grateful for.

45. Watch something funny.

46. Do crafts.

47. Organize your closet.

48. Plan your next holiday gifts.

49. Look up old friends on Facebook or LinkedIn.

50. Make a list like this for yourself.

Appendix 2: Serenity Prayer

Grant me the serenity to accept the things I cannot change, the courage to change the things I can, and the wisdom to know the difference.

Appendix 3: The Un-Less Prayer and Mantra

The Un-Less Prayer

I choose to nourish myself, through my principles and actions. Health begins with heal. I am healing myself because I deserve more, not less. I am lovely. I love me, unconditionally, now.

The Un-Less Mantra

Unconditional Love

Try matching "unconditional" with your inhale and "love" with your exhale for a simple concentrative meditation.

Appendix 4: Other Resources

Many other writers in the world of wellness have inspired me. Here are just a few, each listed with one of his or her greatest books.

1. Geneen Roth, author of *When Food is Love*, on healing poor body image.
2. Andrew Weill, MD, author of *Eating Well to Optimize Health*, on nutrition and Integrative Medicine.
3. Christiane Northrup, MD, author of *Women's Bodies, Women's Wisdom,* on women's health and tuning into your own body.
4. 4. Brian Wansink, author of *Mindless Eating: Why We Eat More Than We Think*, on research about what cues and practices affect intake.
5. Mireille Guilano, author of *French Women Don't Get Fat*, on French cultural norms that do not center on extreme beliefs and allow for healthy indulgence and balance.
6. Mary Pipher, author of *Reviving Ophelia, Saving the Lives of Adolescent Girls*, on deconstructing cultural beliefs that are damaging to young women.
7. Joan Ryan, author of *Little Girls in Pretty Boxes*, on how damaging body norms can be in the world of gymnastics, figure skating, and other competitive sports.
8. Michael Pollan, author of *Omnivore's Dilemma*, on how different foods are sourced and their impact on the environment and our health.